Thoracic Radiology

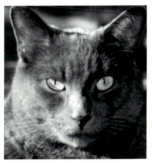

for the Small Animal Practitioner

by Robert T. O'Brien
DVM, MS

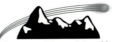

Teton NewMedia
The Innovative Health Science Publisher
Jackson, Wyoming 83001

Executive Editor: Carroll C. Cann

Development Editor: Susan L. Hunsberger

Editor: Cynthia J. Roantree

Design & Layout: Anita B. Sykes

Printer: Grand Teton Lithography, Jackson, WY

Teton NewMedia

P.O. Box 4833

125 South King Street

Jackson, WY 83001

1-888-770-3165

www.tetonnm.com

Radiographs are reproduced with permission from the University of Wisconsin (unless otherwise noted)

Illustrations by Anne Rains

PRINTED IN THE UNITED STATES OF AMERICA

ISBN # 1-893441-08-3

Print number 5 4 3 2 1

        Library of Congress Cataloging-in-Publication Data
O'Brien, Robert T., DVM
    Thoracic radiology for the small animal practitioner / Robert T. O'Brien.
    p. cm.
    Includes bibliographical references.
    ISBN 1-893441-08-3
    1. Veterinary radiography. 2. Dogs--Diseases--Diagnosis. 3.
Cats--Diseases--Diagnosis. 4. Chest--Radiography. I. Title.
    SF757.8.027 2000
    636.7'089607572--dc21

                                                            00-060745

Dedication

To family and friends who inspired me.
To Mo, for your eternal patience and support.

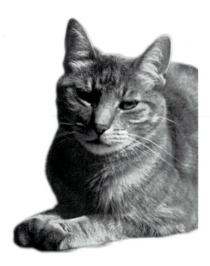

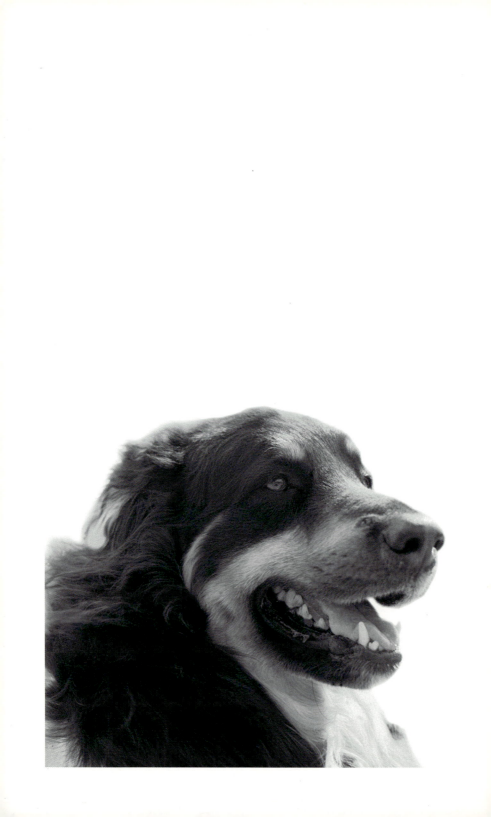

Preface

The detection of thoracic disease is exceptionally challenging. Without the ability to palpate internal structures, imaging takes on a more important role. The clinical evaluation of a coughing dog or dyspneic cat would not be complete without radiology.

The intent of this effort is to provide a high quality convenient manual. The subject matter is derived from many sources. The most important source is the author's own professional experiences as a small animal clinician and radiologist.

We all begin our radiology careers by looking hopelessly at an incomprehensible assortment of black and white dots. Later we falsely find evidence of abnormalities on every image. The real goal is to be able to correctly differentiate variations of normal from real indicators of disease.

This book should assist you by providing a non-threatening resource but it is not all inclusive. I firmly believe that the typical competent small animal clinician is lost with an all-inclusive list of differential diagnoses. What most of us really need is a "reasonable" list of two or three diagnoses. This text makes great effort to limit the differentials to a short practical prioritized list. I hope that this book will help the animal practitioner and aspiring veterinary student to approach radiology with interest and confidence.

Robert T. O'Brien

Table Of Contents

Section 1 Radiology

Section 2 Normal Radiographic Anatomy

Section 3 Radiology of the Heart

Section 4 Vessels

Section 5 Lungs

Section 6 Pleural Space Disease

Section 7 Mediastinum

Section 8 Diaphragm

Section 9 Body Wall and Ribs

Appendices

Recommended Readings

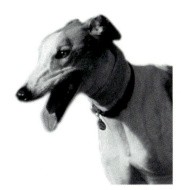

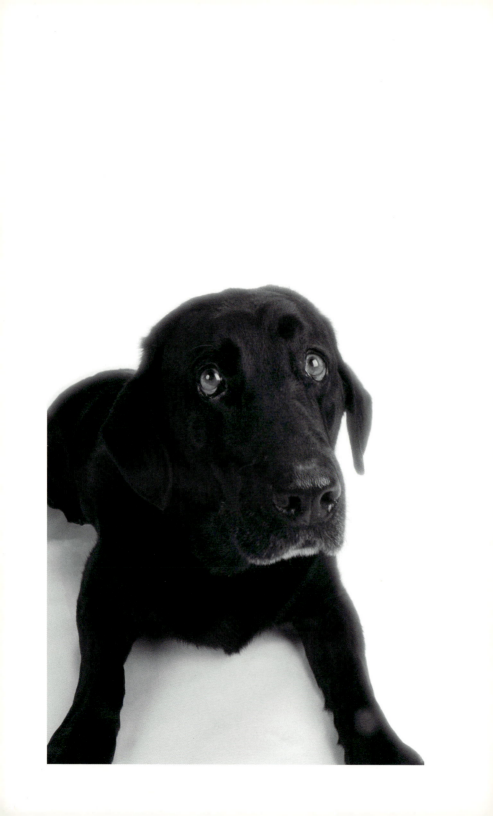

Section 1

Radiography

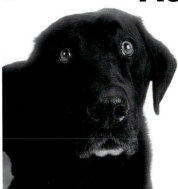

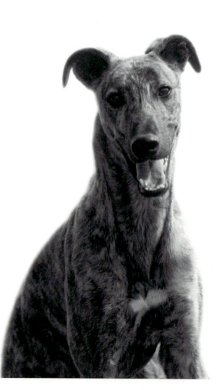

Introduction

The goals of this book are to provide you with the techniques of radiography and radiology of the dog and cat thorax. Thoracic radiology remains the main imaging modality in the interpretation of pulmonary and other intrathoracic diseases.

These techniques should provide you with a basis for producing diagnostic images and interpreting them to derive a reasonable set of differential diagnoses.

Some Helpful Hints

Scattered throughout the text are the following symbols to help you focus on what is really important.

✓   This is a routine feature of the subject being discussed. I've tried to narrow them down.

♥   This is an important feature. You should remember this.

⚷ Critical feature. It is a key to understanding radiography.

✋   Stop. This doesn't look important but it can really make a difference when trying to sort out unusual situations. It can be my opinion based on personal experience.

⊙   A CD is available as an accompaniment to this printed volume. The CD-ROM allows you to search and retrieve the full text, figures, and tables of the book, plus additional artwork. To purchase this CD-ROM, please call 877-306-9793.

Applications of Thoracic Radiology

Applications include:

♥ Characterization of lung disease.

♥ Staging of heart failure.

♥ Staging of metastatic cancer.

✓ Useful in diagnosing dogs and cats with:

    Coughing

    Dyspnea

    Wheezing

    Heart murmur

    Palpable mass

    Severe trauma (hit by a car, etc.)

    Chest wounds

    Vomiting/regurgitation

    Cyanosis

✓ Pre-anesthetic work-up

✓ Suspected electrocution or severe neck trauma

✓ Geriatric screening

Limitations of Thoracic Radiology

⚷ Radiographs provide information, not answers.

✓ Answers are derived from proper interpretation of the radiographic signs in concert with other clinical aspects of the case.

✓ Radiographs may lead you to ask more or different types of clinical questions.

✓ Radiographs of poor quality are a waste of personnel time and client money.

✓ Without a systematic approach to film interpretation, the information may be on the radiograph, but goes unseen.

✓ Without a good knowledge of clinical medicine, changes are noted on the radiographs but incorrect conclusions are reached.

4

Public Health Message

☠ Radiation is HAZARDOUS. Don't risk your health with poor technique.

✓ Repeating radiographs is a common source of unnecessary radiation exposure.

✓ Always collimate the primary x-ray beam.

✓ Collimate to the smaller of these two: the size of the cassette or body size of interest (because scatter radiation from irradiated parts outside the area of interest degrades the image).

✓ Stay outside the room if at all possible.

✓ If clinically necessary to manually restrain the patient, do not have a human body part in the collimated field (EVEN IN LEAD!)

Medical–Legal Issues

Radiographs are a diagnostic medical legal document which should properly identify the patient, date, and clinic name. Patient positioning should be marked (lateral views are marked by the side closest to the cassette) along with anatomic sidedness (left versus right).

What is a Radiograph?

♥ Radiographs are images on photographic film made by x-rays that have passed through tissue. The interaction of x-ray photons with the intensifying screen in the cassette produces photons of visible light. The light interacts with silver in the film to produce a latent image. The latent image is converted into the black and white by the developing process (Figure 1-1).

✓ The whiteness of the film is termed "opacity." There are five radiographic opacities:

    Metal

    Mineral (bone)

    Soft tissue (water, blood)

    Fat

    Air

✓ The resultant opacity of the image is a function of both the object density and the thickness of the structure (which is why some end-on blood vessels can appear as opaque as a rib).

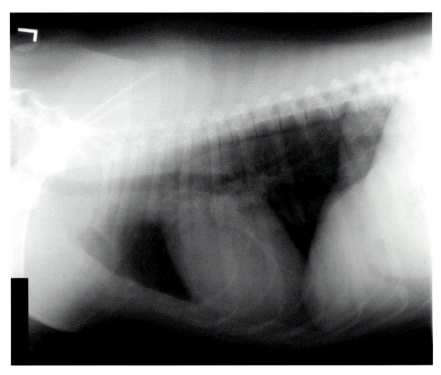

Figure 1-1
Normal 2 year old female spayed Labrador retriever. Note distinct borders of scapula and spinous processes of cranial thoracic vertebrae.

✔ The film has characteristics that allow us to image structures as varied as air-filled objects to metallic objects on the same radiograph.

✔ We depend on proper technique, positioning, and accurate developing for the production of diagnostic images.

A Brief Discussion of Film Artifacts

♥ Artifacts are misrepresentations of real objects or an image of something not real.

✔ Artifacts are a subject requiring a clever eye and detective's insight.

✔ This discussion will be limited to a simple means of interpretation.

   Too much blackness or discrete black marks are too many silver granules converted to visible blackness and is termed "film fog". It is usually caused by the application of pressure (bending the film), chemicals (water, extraneous processing chemicals), electricity (static electricity), or heat. Generalized blackness can be due to overdeveloping or over exposure.

White marks mean too few silver granules converted to visible blackness and are caused by

interruption of photons to the film from dirt or foreign material on the collimator, the patient's skin, or the table top, or the grid improperly aligned with the path of the x-ray beam.

incomplete conversion of x-ray energy to light energy (bad screens).

incomplete conversion of silver in the latent image to crystalline silver (under developing).

Blurring is caused by

patient motion (slow technique); high "S" part of the milliamp x seconds (mAs).

penumbra (normal divergence of the x-ray beam after penetrating the body part)

incomplete apposition of the film and screens (not closed tightly or broken)

double exposure

Thoracic Radiography

✓ Any weak link in the chain of positioning, technique, or developing can lead to a nondiagnostic image.

✓ If you are hand-developing, remember that your chemicals need regular maintenance and to use time-temperature developing, not guesswork or experience.

✓ If you want consistent high-quality radiographs with minimal maintenance, purchase an automatic processor.

✓ Use rare earth screens.

✓ Use a grid with bigger patients (greater than 10 cm thick).

Positioning

🖐 The diagnostic value of a radiograph is more dependent on positioning than any other single factor (Figures 1-2 and 1-3). Refer to the Appendix for positioning techniques.

✔ Remove all foreign objects—collars, leashes, bandages, dirt, water, or blood.

✔ Restrain the patient either chemically or physically. Restraint techniques are limited by clinical concerns and patient compliance.

✔ Clever use of sandbags, rope, tape, and straps minimizes the radiation dose to holders.

✔ The front legs should be pulled forward so that they are not superimposed on the chest.

✔ On ventrodorsal or dorsoventral (VD/DV) views, the spine MUST be superimposed on the sternum.

✔ On lateral projections, elevation of the sternum is often necessary so that the sternum and spine are the same distance above the cassette.

Interpretation of Positioning

Features of the Properly Positioned Lateral Projection

✔ Ribs extend equally and are parallel

✔ Costal arches do not extend more ventral than the sternum (except symmetrically as a breed variant)

✔ Ribs do not extend more dorsal than the spine (unless symmetrically)

Features of the Properly Positioned VD/DV

🖐 Sternum is superimposed on the spine throughout the entire length of the thorax.

✔ The ribs are symmetrical in shape and the spine is in a straight line.

What Views Do I Take?

🖐 Enough to provide the complete set of information.

🖐 Typical studies include 3 views: left and right lateral, and VD views.

✔ Opposite laterals provide better detection for focal diseases (lobar pneumonia and nodules) (Figures 1-4, 1-5, and 1-6).

✔ The VD view "opens" the chest, providing better lung disease detection.

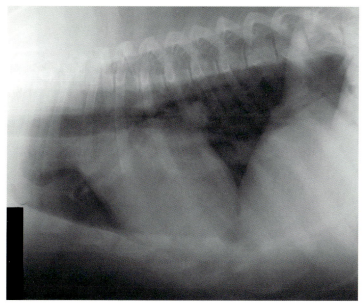

Figure 1-2
Normal 4 year old male neutered Newfoundland. Note the increased opacity in heart base due to the oblique angle.

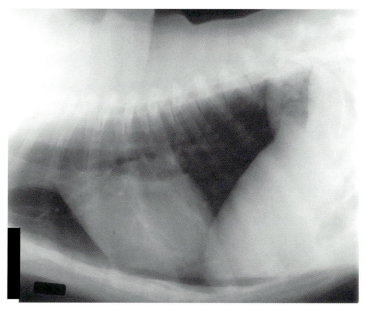

Figure 1-3
Normal 4 year old male neutered Newfoundland. Note more normal appearance of heart base region.

✔ The VD view is indicated with suspected pleural effusion.

✔ For 99.9% of disease detection, inspiratory-phase radiographs are indicated.

✔ Inspiration provides the best biological contrast between the air-filled lung and soft tissue opacity disease (pneumonia, nodules, etc.).

Exceptions

✔ The DV view provides a better view of the heart base and caudal lobar vessels.

🖐 The DV view may be better tolerated by dyspneic patients, especially cats.

✔ In severely dyspneic patients:

Be judicious and efficient.

Premeasure the patient before transport to radiology.

Set the machine technique and gown up before bringing the patient in.

Position the cassette and collimate the beam before the patient arrives.

Perhaps take only one view–a lateral view is the least stressful.

♥ Maybe wait until tomorrow: patients should not die while you attempt a diagnostic procedure.

♥ Expiratory-phase radiographs

✔ Detection of:

♥ Gas filled masses (bullae)

♥ Collapsing intrathoracic trachea and main stem bronchi (See Section 7)

Technique

Technique refers to the balance of kVp and mAs. You want a high kVp-low mAs technique. Interpreting a film that is a little too gray is easier than one that is too black and white (Figures 1-7 and 1-8). Low mAs mean a very short exposure time, which will stop the breathing motion. The thorax has very high contrast inherently and can withstand a high kVp.

A technique chart should be constructed for all species and body parts imaged (See Appendix A). It is based on the maximum dimension, usually at the level of the last rib. The chart can be made from a standing or recumbent patient, but if the chart was made from a recumbent patient, measure for radiology in recum-

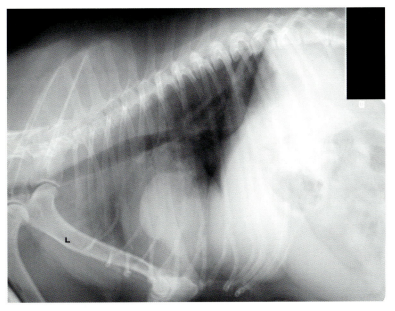

Figure 1-4
Left lateral projection of 12 year old female spayed Schnauzer with large mass in right middle lung lobe. Mass was a primary lung neoplasia.

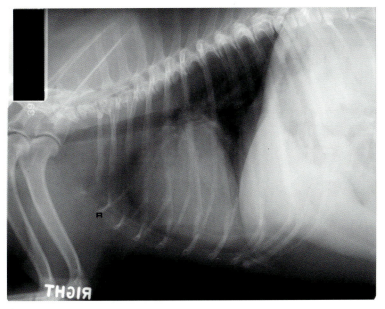

Figure 1-5
Same dog as in Figure 1-4. Mass can no longer be seen in the right lateral projection when the mass is in the dependent lung lobe.

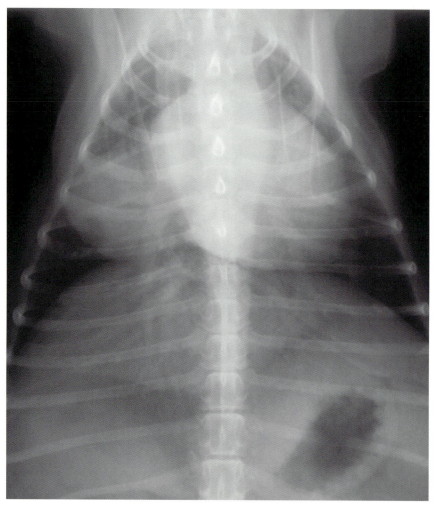

Figure 1-6
Same dog as Figure 1-4. Mass is seen in the right middle lung lobe.

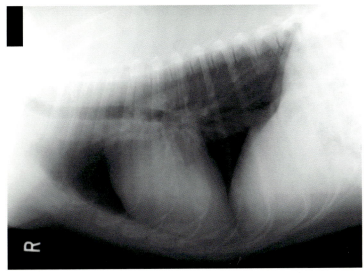

Figure 1-7
Normal 2 year old female spayed Labrador Retriever using high kVp and low mAs technique. Note ability to see spine of scapula through vertebral bodies, liver margins, and pulmonary vessels in lung periphery.

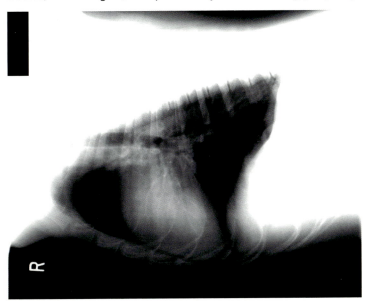

Figure 1-8
Same dog as Figure 1-7 with much more contrast. This usually is a result of low kVp technique. Note inability to see distinct margins of bone structures and organs in the abdomen. The more lucent areas of the lung are too black to view with routine lighting on a view box and require a bright light.

bency. Be consistent. Inaccurate measurements invalidate the technique chart, ensuring poor quality radiographs.

Film Reading Technique

🖐 Learn a system, then use it!

🖐 Look at the ENTIRE film.

✓ My system is listed below but any system used consistently is a good system

✓ Study the peripheral structures in a clockwise direction starting cranially:

> Forelimb
>
> Neck (soft tissues, spine and trachea)
>
> Thoracic spine (spinous processes, spinal canal, and vertebral bodies)
>
> Diaphragm
>
> Stomach
>
> Liver (and any other visible intra-abdominal structure)
>
> Falciform fat pad and other intra-abdominal fat
>
> Sternum

Next study the mediastinum and pleural spaces, the ribs for symmetry (turn the VD/DV film upside down to better detect rib fractures), the heart, and the lungs.

Look at the dark areas: inevitably, there will be overexposed portions on every film; so purchase a bright light. To increase acuity in detecting lesions in the darker area of the film, I use two lightly clenched hands arranged in a series (Figure 1-9) or an empty paper towel roll (Figure 1-10). Both of these limit the extraneous light and allow you to concentrate on the body portion to be evaluated.

Two definitions that will help in interpreting radiographs are **silhouette** and **summation**.

1. **Silhouette:** Two objects of the same opacity that touch each other lose their margins. Examples include free pleural fluid surrounding the heart and the alveolar lung pattern (pus-filled alveoli touching the serosal border of bronchi).

2. **Summation:** Two objects that do not touch but are along the same x-ray path cause the resultant image to be the sum of both opacities.

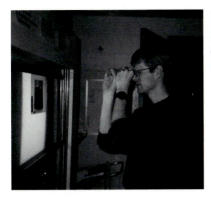

Figure 1-9
Demonstration of limiting extraneous light with two clenched hands (Bob-o-scope).

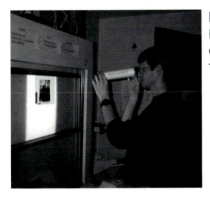

Figure 1-10
Demonstration of limiting extraneous light with opaque tube.

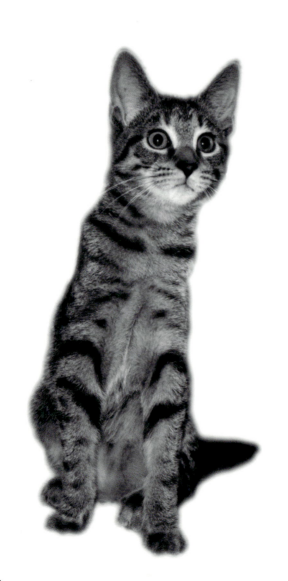

Normal Radiographic Anatomy

Introduction

☛ Knowledge of what is considered "normal" is essential for detecting lesions.

🖐 "Normal" includes all the variations by age, breed, sex, and body condition.

🖐 Radiographic variations are as clinically important as, and more difficult to learn, than normal radiographic anatomy (Figures 2-1, 2-2, and 2-3 and 2-4).

🖐 Cats are not little dogs.

Radiologic Variations
Patient Positioning

🖐 Expiration causes increased lung opacity. Decreased amount of air in the lungs results in proportional increased interstitial pattern (see Figures 5-1 and 5-2). Overlap of the diaphragm and caudal cardiac silhouette should alert you to this variation. (see Obesity)

🖐 Underexposure causes increased lung opacity. Poor penetration of the spine, especially superimposed on the scapula, should alert you to this variation. This is a common problem with obese patients if the technique is not adjusted accordingly.

✔ Flexion of the neck causes bending of the trachea in the lateral projection. Undulation of the trachea should not be mistaken for "dorsal deviation" secondary to a cranial mediastinal mass. Repeating the radiograph with the neck hyperextended tests the validity of the tracheal positioning due to head position.

✔ Rotation of the chest in the lateral projection makes the heart base appear larger (see Figure 1-2). Without foam support beneath the ventrum, an increased opacity in the heart base mimics left atrium enlargement and hilar lymphadenopathy.

✔ Oblique positioning on VD/DV projections distorts the cardiac silhouette mimicking chamber enlargements.

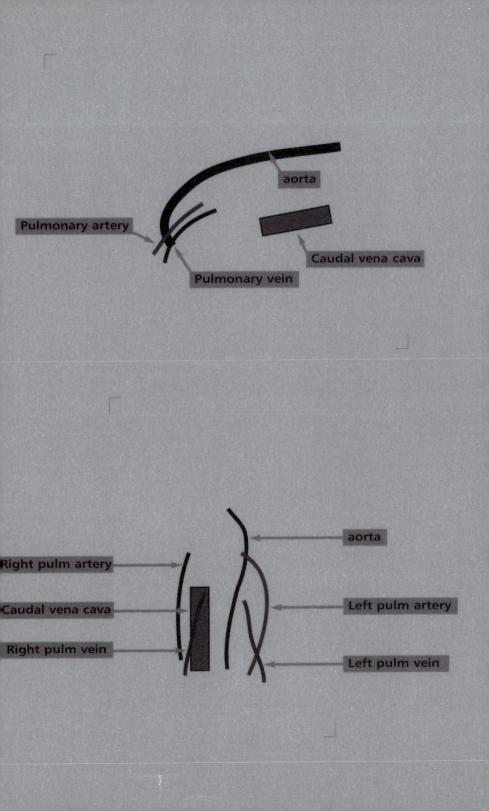

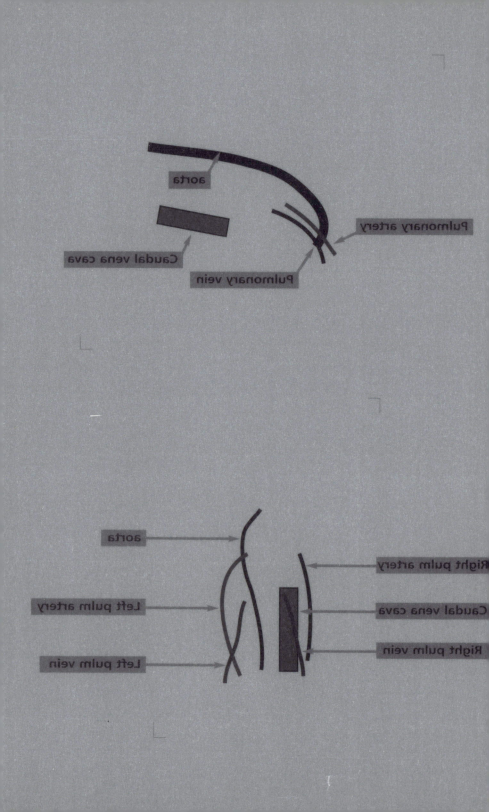

aorta

Caudal vena cava

Pulmonary vein

Pulmonary artery

aorta

Right pulm artery

Left pulm artery

Caudal vena cava

Left pulm vein

Right pulm vein

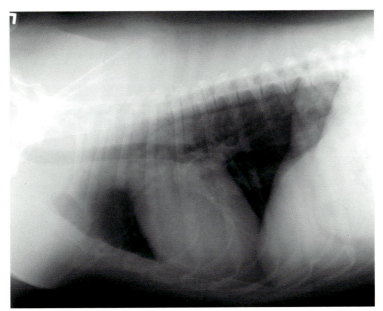

Figure 2-1
Normal 2 year old female spayed Labrador Retriever lateral view.

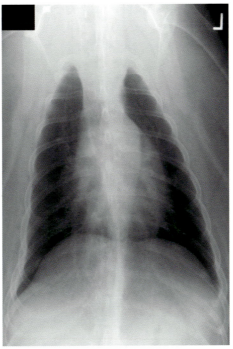

Figure 2-2.
Normal 11 year old female spayed Alaskan malamute, ventrodorsal view.

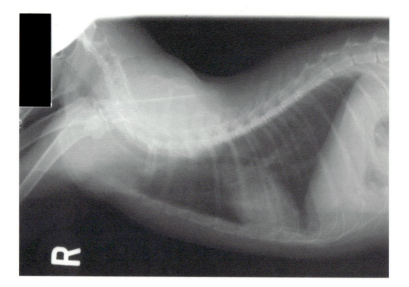

Figure 2-3
Normal 5 year old female spayed domestic short-haired cat, lateral view

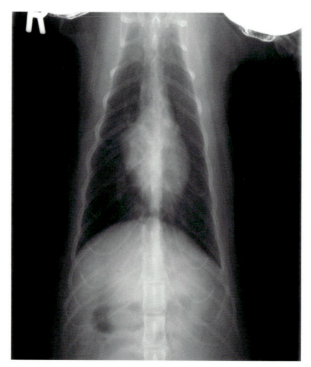

Figure 2-4
Same cat as Figure 2-3, ventrodorsal view.

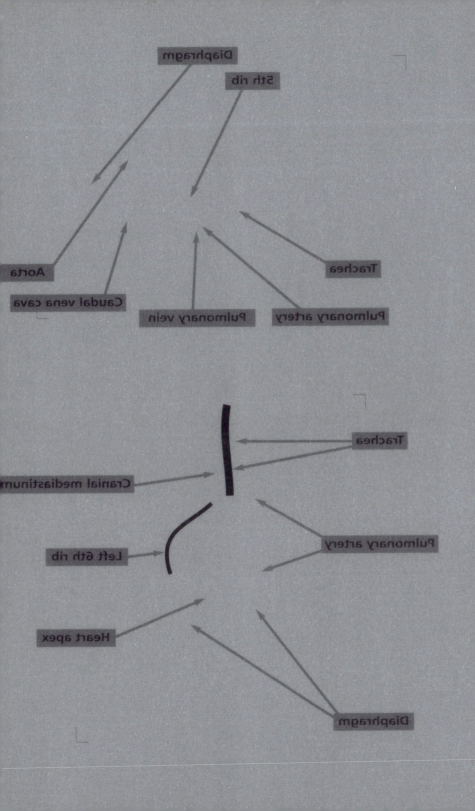

Diaphragm

5th rib

Aorta

Caudal vena cava

Pulmonary vein

Pulmonary artery

Trachea

Trachea

Cranial mediastinum

Left 6th rib

Pulmonary artery

Heart apex

Diaphragm

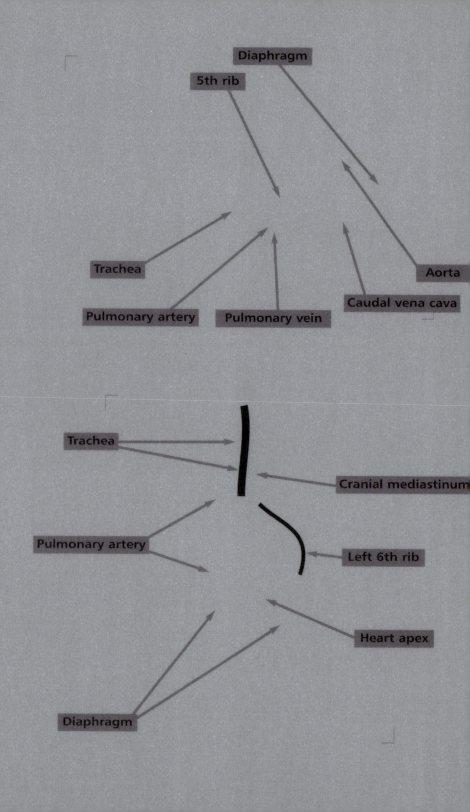

Diaphragm

5th rib

Trachea

Pulmonary artery

Pulmonary vein

Caudal vena cava

Aorta

Trachea

Cranial mediastinum

Pulmonary artery

Left 6th rib

Heart apex

Diaphragm

Geriatric Patients

Variations in geriatric patients include:

🖐 Increased lung opacity. This is mostly due to combined increased bronchial and interstitial patterns. The bronchial pattern is caused by dystrophic mineralization in the walls. The interstitial component is thought to be due to pulmonary fibrosis in cats and dogs (Figures 2-5, 2-6 and 2-7).

✓ Mineralized costal cartilages (cats and dogs).

✓ Mineralized costochondral junctions. Often exuberant, this change is an incidental finding. It is more common in dogs.

✓ Spondylosis deformans. This radiographic change (more common in dogs) is associated with smooth bone formation extending from the vertebral end plates toward the adjacent vertebral end plate. This change is thought to be a degeneration of the annulus fibrosis part of the intervertebral disk and, as an isolated finding, can be considered incidental (see Figure 2-5).

✓ Heart orientation: The heart in older animals (more common in cats) tends to be less upright (it "falls forward" or "leans over") than in young animals. This exaggerates the appearance of the aortic arch on both the lateral and VD/DV views (see Figures 2-6 and 2-7).

✓ Thickening of pleural fissures due to fibrosis may mimic pleural effusion.

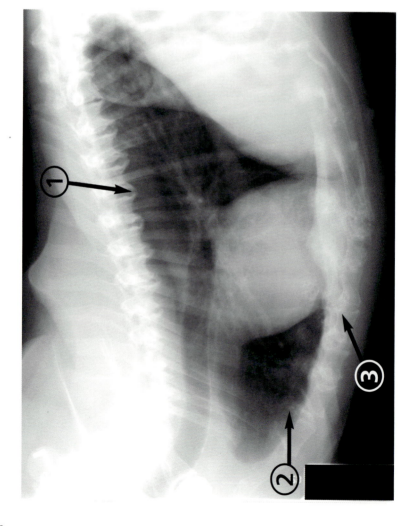

Figure 2-5

Normal geriatric 13 year old.female spayed German shepherd. Note spondylosis deformans of thoracic spine (1), mineralized costochondral junctions (2), degenerative changes in sternebral junctions (3), and generalize increased bronchointerstitial lung pattern.

22

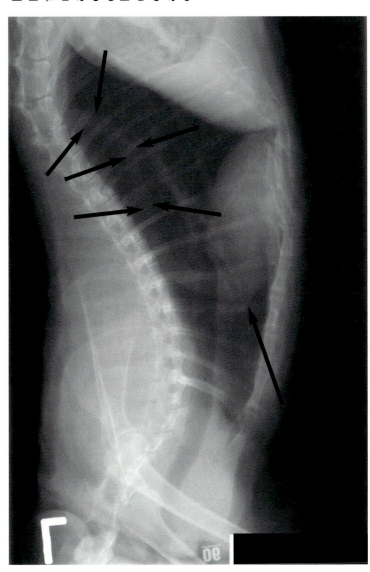

Figure 2-6
Normal 8 year old female spayed Siamese mix cat. Note the apparent increased size of aortic arch (arrows) due to more horizontal heart orientation. Note undulating appearance of descending aorta and mineralized costal cartilages.

23

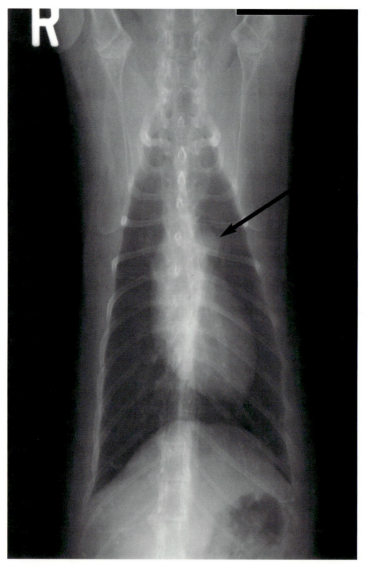

Figure 2-7
View showing apparent increased size of aortic arch (arrow).

Obesity

Variations caused by obesity are:

🖐 Increased lung opacity. This is mostly due to an increased interstitial pattern that is caused by relative expiration. The weight of the thoracic wall fat limits chest wall excursions, and intra-abdominal fat decreases the caudal movement of the diaphragm. Increase the kVp 10% to 15% compared to a patient of normal conformation of the same measurements. (Figures 2-8, 2-9, 2-10, and 2-11).

🖐 Apparent increased heart size. The smaller lung volume makes the heart appear larger (out of proportion). This is a challenge when using both the subjective interpretation and a cardiac measuring scheme that uses intercostal spaces or percent of chest width.

🖐 Increased width of the mediastinum. Fat infiltration in the cranial mediastinum can mimic a mass in cats and dogs. This increased width usually has parallel sides, as seen on the VD/DV view, unlike a mass. In the middle mediastinum, the fat adjacent to the heart may silhouette with the cardiac outline mimicking heart enlargement. Caudal mediastinal widening between the accessory and caudal left lung lobes can be mistaken for pleural effusion.

🖐 The fat adjacent to the heart in cats can be very difficult to differentiate from cardiac enlargement. A lower kVp (65-70) and higher mAs technique may allow detection of the soft tissue (heart)-fat border.

🖐 Increased distance between lung lobes or between lung and inner body wall. Fat can accumulate in pleural fissures or on the inner aspect of the chest wall, mimicking pleural effusion.

Breed Variations

✓ Brachycephalic dogs have smaller diameter of trachea than normal. Other brachycephalic breeds (Boxers, Boston Bulldogs) are smaller than normal and English Bulldogs are smaller yet. Apparently larger heart size is a result of wide shallow conformation.

✓ Any patient with loose skin (cats or dogs) may mimic pneumothorax on VD/DV projection.

🖐 Bulldogs: A Bulldog is not a Bulldog without a caudal thoracic hemivertebra (Figures 2-12 and 2-13).

🖐 Dachshunds and Greyhounds have hearts that measure big using the Vertebral Heart Scale

✓ Collies commonly have heterotopic bone formation in the lungs which mimic metastatic nodules (Figure 2-14).

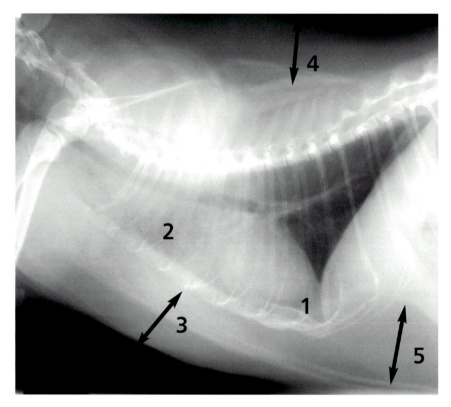

Figure 2-8
Obese 15 year old male neutered domestic short-hair cat. Note increased opacity in caudoventral (1) and cranial (2) lung fields. The cranial cardiac border is indistinct. Increased fat is seen in the ventral (3) and dorsal (4) bodywalls, and in the falciform region (5).

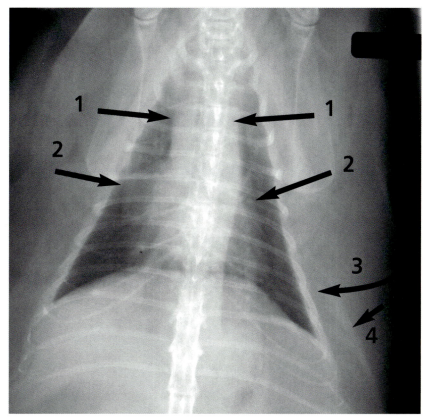

Figure 2-9
Same cat as Figure 2-8. Increased width of the cranial mediastinum (1), apparent increased width of the cardiac silhouette (2), increased amount of subcutaneous fat in the body wall (3), and increased opacity of fascial planes of bodywall musculature (4) can be seen.

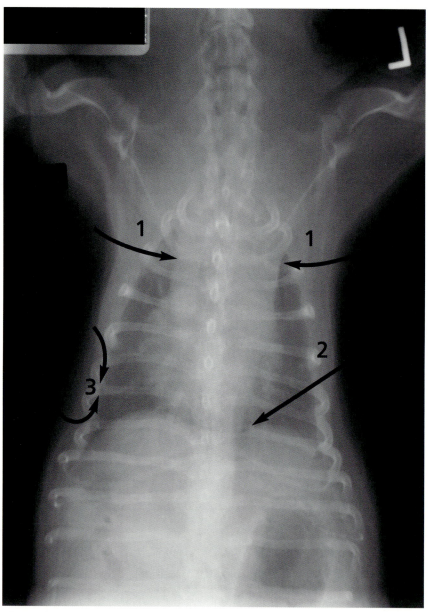

Figure 2-10

Obese 15 year old male Pekinese. This view shows increased width of the cranial mediastinum (1), the increased overlap of heart and diaphragm (2), and the fat within the pleural space (3) mimicking pleural effusion.

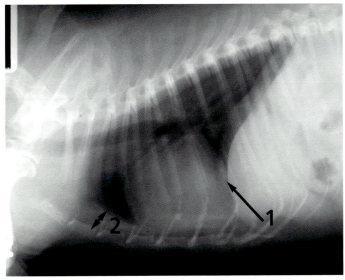

Figure 2-11
Same dog as Figure 2-8. The increased overlap of heart and diaphragm (1) give the impression of increased heart size. Fat within the mediastinal and pleural spaces (2) mimics pleural effusion.

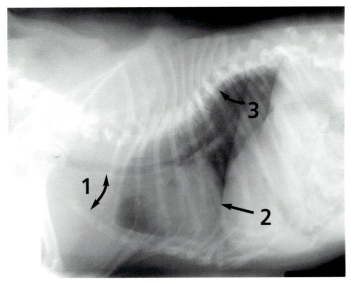

Figure 2-12
Normal 2 year old male neutered English Bulldog. Note increased height of cranial mediastinum (1), overlap of heart and diaphragm (2), and hemivertebra (3).

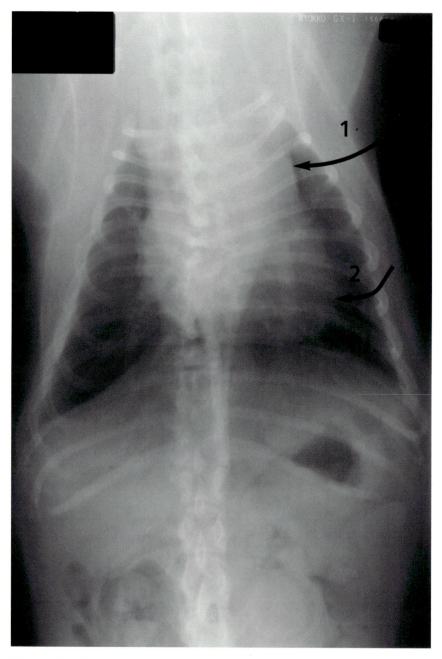

Figure 2-13
Same Bulldog as Figure 2-12. This view shows the increased width of cranial mediastinum (1), and the shift of the cardiac apex to the left (2).

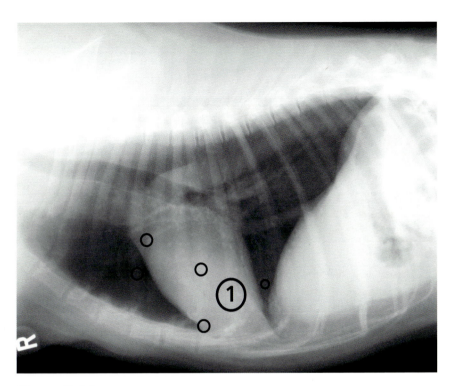

Figure 2-14
Normal 13 year old male neutered Collie with heterotopic bone in the lungs (1).

Body Wall Variations

✓ Skin folds (see Figure 3-14)

✓ Nipples, ticks, dirt, and costochondral junctions may mimic pulmonary nodules (Figure 2-15).

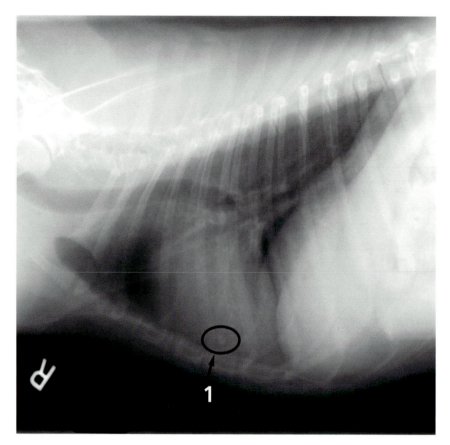

Figure 2-15
Normal 7 year old female spayed English Pointer dog with nipple (1) superimposed on the lungs mimicking a pulmonary mass.

Section 3

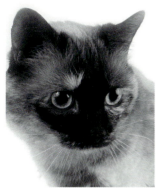

Radiology of the Heart

☞ This is the first section on radiology because it is the first organ in my radiologic method (see previous). It is also first because the heart is inherently important as a body system. I prefer to evaluate the heart before the lungs. Heart disease more often leads to secondary lung changes than primary lung disease causes secondary heart problems.

Techniques

✔ As mentioned previously, it is essential to get at least two views of the heart.

✔ On the VD view, the heart will appear longer and narrower than on the DV view.

✋ All dog hearts are more or less in the shape of a reverse "D"—more rounded on the right side in barrel-chested breeds and less so in deep-chested breeds.

✋ Cats have an almond-shaped heart—more slender and fusiform-shaped than dogs.

Evaluation Methods

In this section I describe shape and size criteria of normal hearts in dogs and cats.

✔ Heart size is a complex and somewhat controversial subject. Many clinicians depend on a subjective interpretation, or feeling, which is based on experience with hundreds of radiographs. It is a difficult method to teach.

✔ Regardless of the method used, practice it regularly, even on hearts with obvious changes, to test its sensitivity (how often you call an abnormal heart abnormal).

✔ By practicing on hearts that are obviously normal, you develop a feeling for the method's specificity (how often you call a normal heart normal).

✔ Obviously we would prefer a very sensitive and specific method, but all methods have their flaws.

Method for Detecting Focal Heart Chamber Enlargement in Cats and Dogs

Starting with shape changes, we need to discuss the method to detect focal chamber enlargement.

♥ The best method for detecting focal chamber enlargement, in both dogs and cats, is the clock face method.

Hints on the clock face method:

✔ The analogy considers the outside contour of the heart. It does not section the heart into pie-shaped slices.

✔ The tracheal bifurcation is 12 o'clock on the lateral view.

✔ The cranial midline is 12 o'clock on the VD/DV view.

🖐 The heart apex is 6 o'clock on all views (even if the apex is off midline). Although this results in a somewhat distorted clock, the numbers are easier to remember.

Using these criteria, the clock face analogy is:

Lateral view (Figure 3-1)

12 – 3 o'clock	left atrium
3 – 6 o'clock	left ventricle
6 – 9 o'clock	right ventricle
9 – 12 o'clock	right auricle, aortic arch, and pulmonary trunk

VD/DV view (Figure 3-2)

11 – 1 o'clock	aortic arch
1 – 2 o'clock	main pulmonary artery segment
12 – 3 o'clock	left auricle
3 – 6 o'clock	left ventricle
6 – 9 o'clock	right ventricle
9 – 11 o'clock	right atrium

♥ Note that you need the two projections to evaluate both atria and both auricles.

✔ The apex of the heart is usually on the left of midline in dogs and on the midline in cats.

✔ A cardiac apex to the right of midline bears close examination. However, without other abnormalities, it is a normal variation.

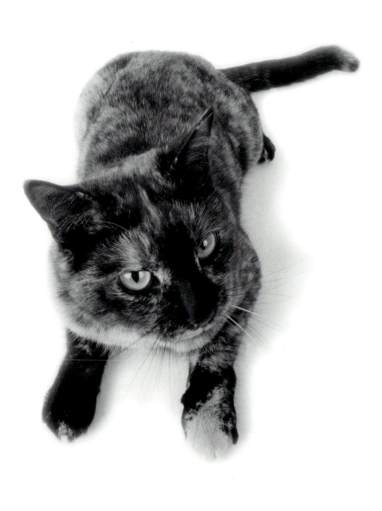

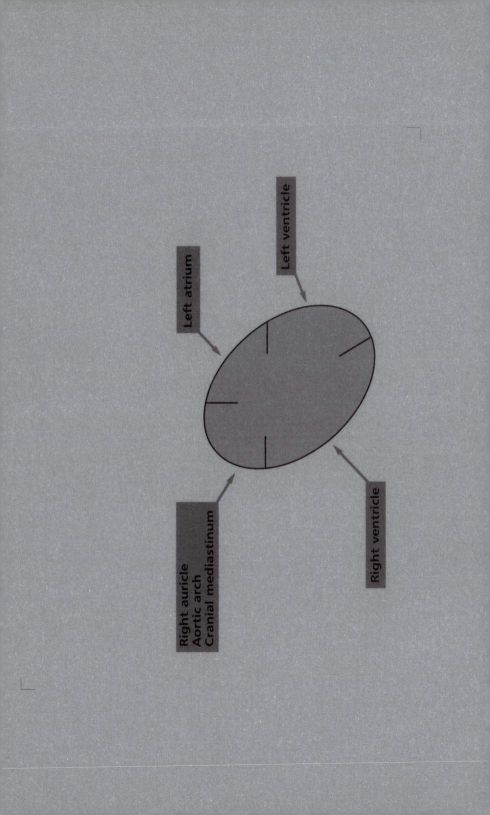

Left atrium

Left ventricle

Right ventricle

Right auricle
Aortic arch
Cranial mediastinum

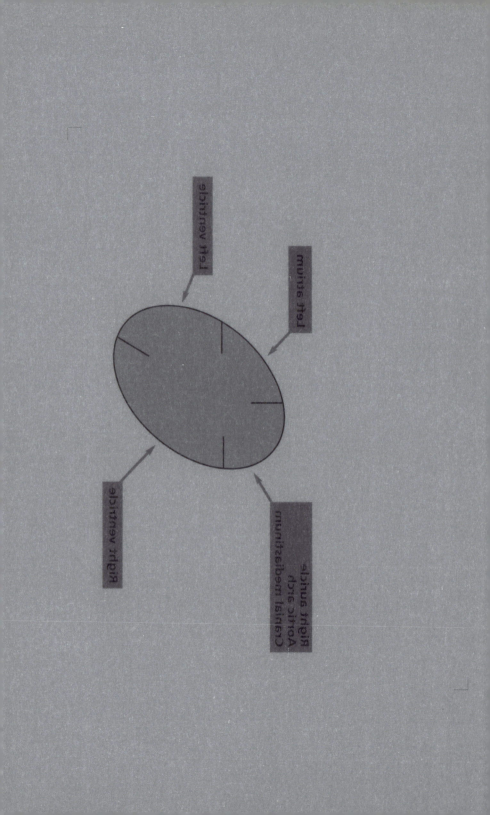

Left ventricle

Left atrium

Right ventricle

Right auricle
Aortic arch
Cranial mediastinum

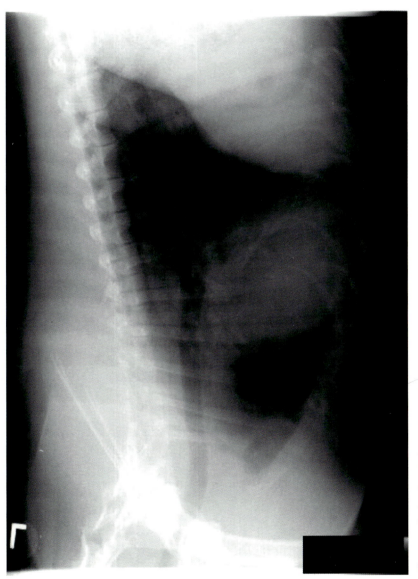

Figure 3-1 Clock face, lateral view

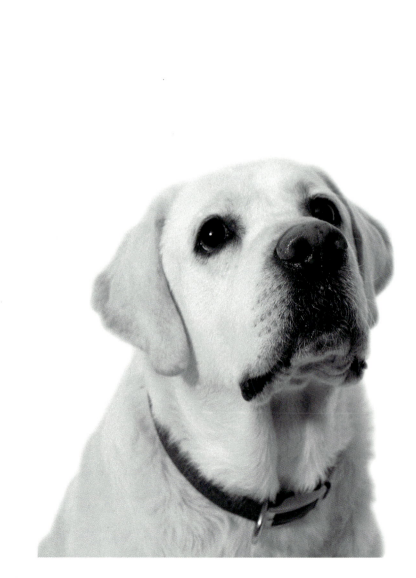

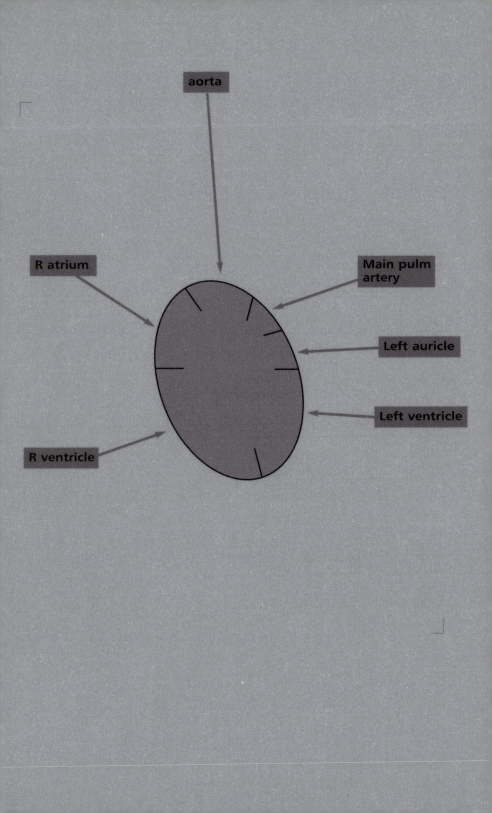

aorta

R atrium

Main pulm
artery

Left auricle

Left ventricle

R ventricle

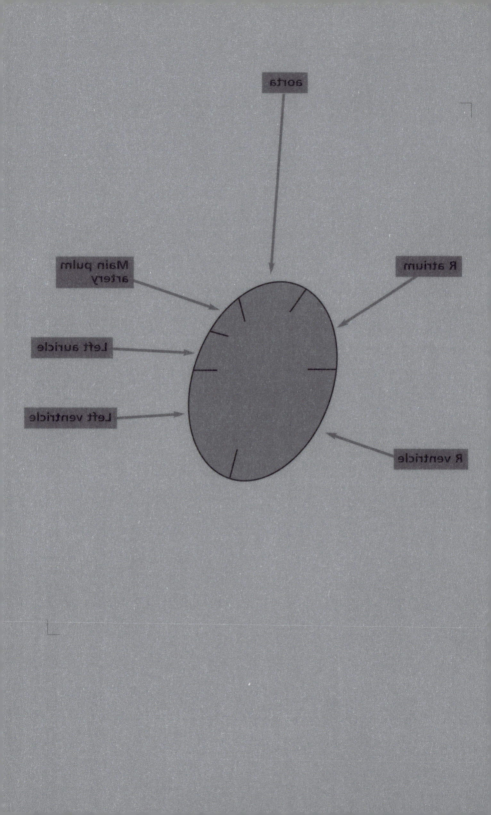

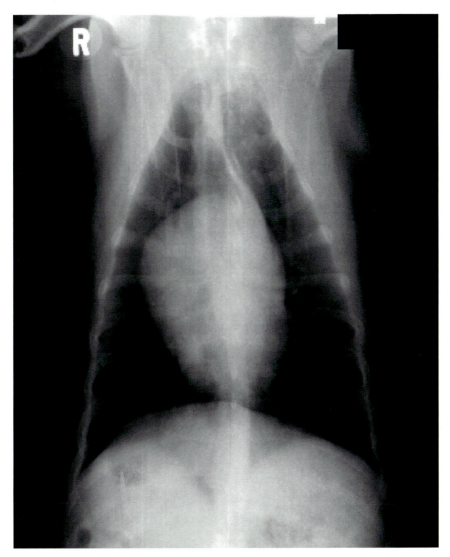

Figure 3-2
Clock face ventrodorsal/dorsoventral view

Methods for Detecting Generalized Heart Enlargement

Dogs

♥ Dogs are easier to evaluate than cats. The best objective system, the Vertebral Heart Scale System (Figure 3-3), works only for dogs.

Proper use of the Vertebral Heart Scale System

1. Using a sheet of paper (not a ruler, pencil, or an estimate), place the leading edge of the paper on the ventral-most aspect of the tracheal bifurcation. Using that as a pivot point, spin the paper so that it is aligned with the longest axis of the heart (base to apex). Mark the location where the tip of the heart apex crosses your paper.

2. Rotate the paper so that it is now 90° to the previous long-axis measurement. The leading edge (same as the long axis) of the paper will be on the cranial margin of the heart. Slide the paper up or down the long axis until you find the widest part of the heart. Again mark the caudal border of the heart.

3. Be very careful to measure the width perpendicular to the long axis, not along the horizontal plane. If you measure along the horizontal plane (parallel to the long axis of the dog) most hearts will measure big, making the method seem very nonspecific.

4. Move your paper so that the leading edge is now superimposed over the cranial-most aspect of the body of the 4th thoracic vertebra. Align the paper so that it is parallel to the spine. Count the number of vertebrae for both the length and width. The sum is the heart size expressed in number of vertebrae. Do not try to account for disk space; the system factors that into the equation.

✔ As originally published, the upper limit of normal is 10.5 vertebrae.

🖐 Although this is an excellent method, many normal dogs measure in the 10.5 to 11.0 range. Be cautious with dogs that have no clinical signs. The clinical relevance of a heart that measures large is supporting evidence of suspected cardiac disease, especially heart failure. Treating a normal dog for suspected heart failure is not a minor undertaking. When in doubt, measure again and look for supportive radiographic evidence (vascular congestion, edema, or effusion) or clinical evidence (pulse, ECG, or echocardiographic abnormalities).

🖐 Most dogs, unlike cats, have echocardiographic evidence of the cause of their heart murmur. If you hear a murmur, look hard for the cause.

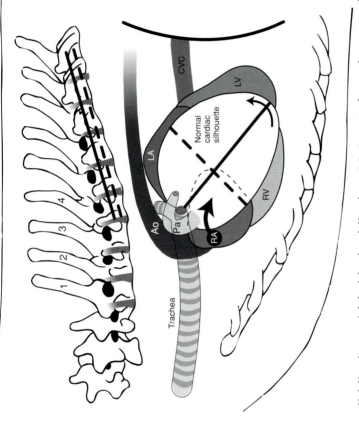

Figure 3-3 Length (solid line) + width (dashed line) = 10.5 vertebrae (=normal) Vertebral heart scale system for dogs and diagrammatic representation of regional heart enlargement.

Cats

✓ Cats are difficult to evaluate. Many attempts have been made to find an objective means of measuring heart size in cats.

🖐 None of them are perfect, but here are some hints.

Lateral view (Figure 3-4):

Width: No wider than two intercostal spaces:

🖐 Does not work well in obese animals or cats with extreme hypoinflated or hyperinflated chests.

Height: Less than 70% the height of the thorax:

🖐 This is difficult to use in elderly cats with tilted hearts. See comment under Width.

VD/DV view (Figure 3-5):

🖐 Width: Half the width of the chest: Influenced by obesity and other diseases.

🖐 No wider than 4 vertebral segments (measured on VD/DV, compared to spine on lateral; see previous dog discussion).

🖐 So what is useful? Width is more important than height, and the DV/VD view is more important than the lateral. Any width, as measured on the VD/DV, that is increased beyond 4 vertebrae and causes rounding of the almond shape should raise your suspicions.

✓ Be cautious. Fat adjacent to the heart can silhouette with the heart, mimicking cardiomegaly in an obese patient.

✓ Use the clock face method. Look for edema, effusion, or congested vessels.

🖐 Be cautious. In cats, 10% to 30% of murmurs are innocent: no cause can be determined on echocardiography or ECG.

Signs of Left-Sided Enlargement

☝ The left is the most common side that is enlarged in cats and dogs and it is very common secondary to mitral valve disease (Figures 3-6 and 3-7).

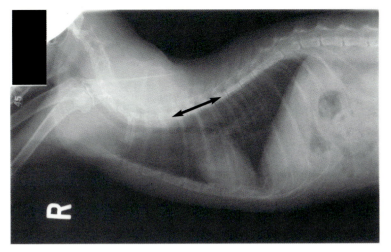

Figure 3-4
Normal cat heart, lateral view (arrow indicates the measurement
taken from the VD view) = 3.5 vertabrae.

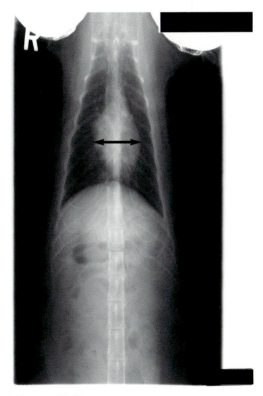

Figure 3-5
Normal cat heart, VD view (arrow indicates maximum heart width).

✓ Cardiomegaly (per verterbral scale system)

✓ Left atrial and ventricular enlargement (per clock face method)

♥ Severe left-sided enlargement can result in generalized cardiomegaly.

⚷ Features of left atrial enlargement

    Lateral projection

        Bulging at 12 to 3 o'clock

        Dorsal displacement of the left caudal lobar bronchus

    VD/DV projection

        Abnormal rounding of the proximal aspect of the caudal lobar arteries ("bow-legged cowboy")

        Increased opacity in the caudal heart base

        Auricular enlargement (2 to 3 o'clock)

⚷ Left ventricular enlargement

    Lateral projection

        A tall heart (combination of left atrial and ventricular enlargement)

        Decreased distance between caudal thoracic trachea and spine (tracheal elevation).

        Rounding at 3 to 6 o'clock

    VD/DV projection

        A long heart

        Rounding at 3 to 6 o'clock

⚷ Concurrent abnormalities

    Increased width of pulmonary veins indicates pulmonary congestion. See Vessels section.

    Pulmonary edema. See Lung section.

    Narrowing of the left caudal lobar bronchus (more easily seen on the lateral view than on the VD/DV view)

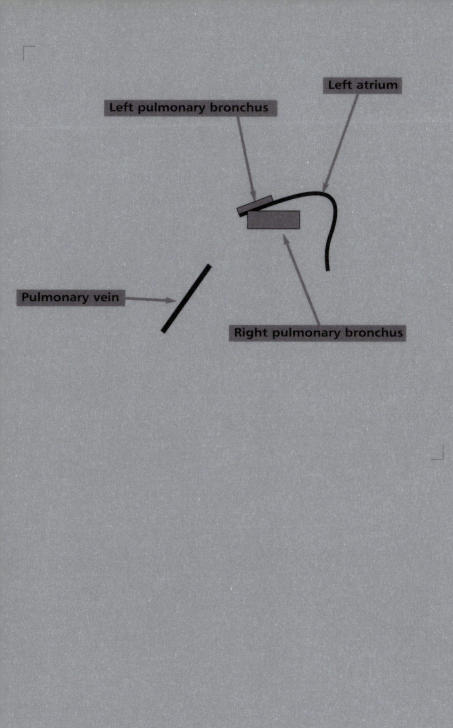

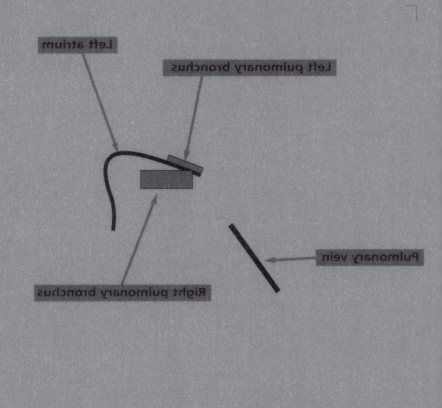

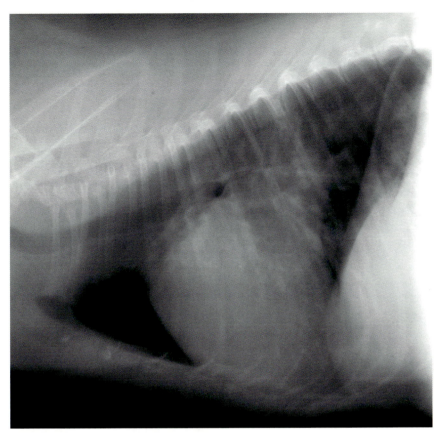

Figure 3-6

A 14 year old female spayed Peekapoo with mitral valve insufficiency secondary to endocardiosis. Note enlargement of left atrium, narrowing of left main stem bronchus, and enlarged pulmonary veins.

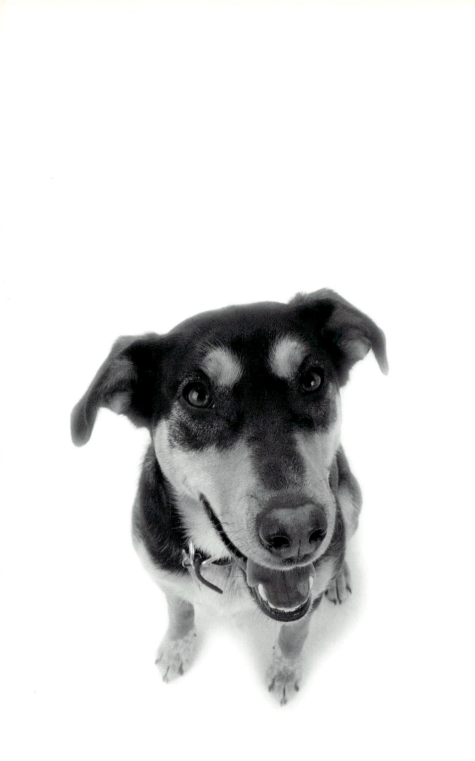

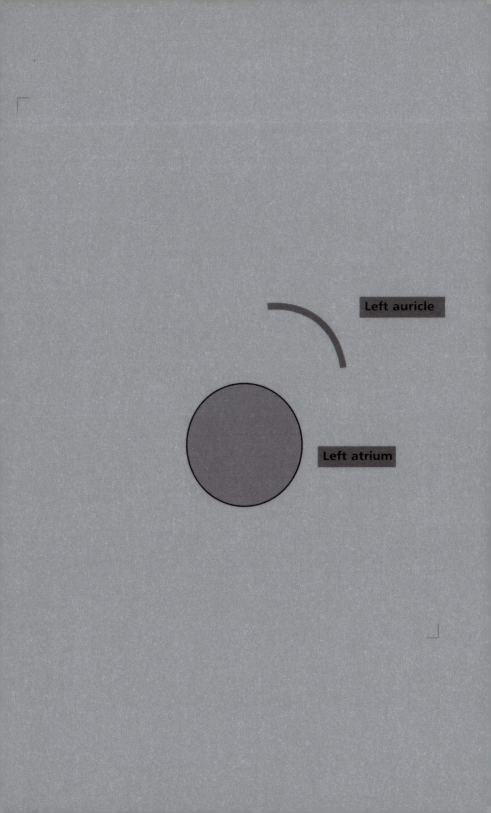

Left auricle

Left atrium

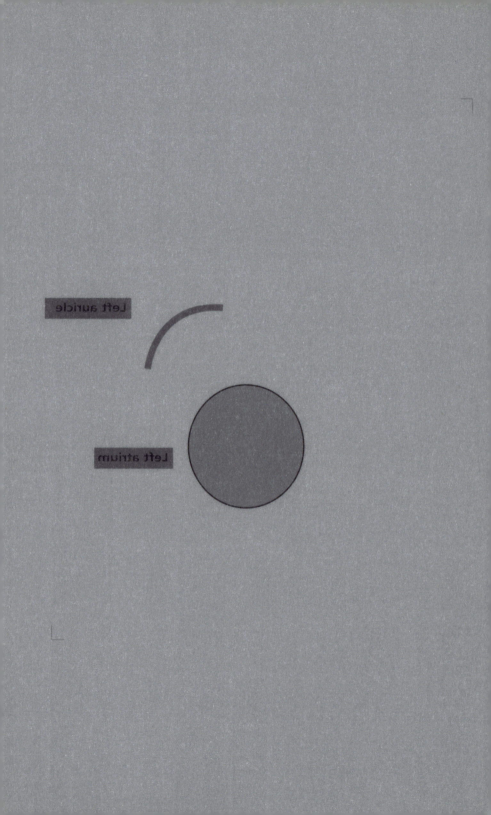

Left auricle

Left atrium

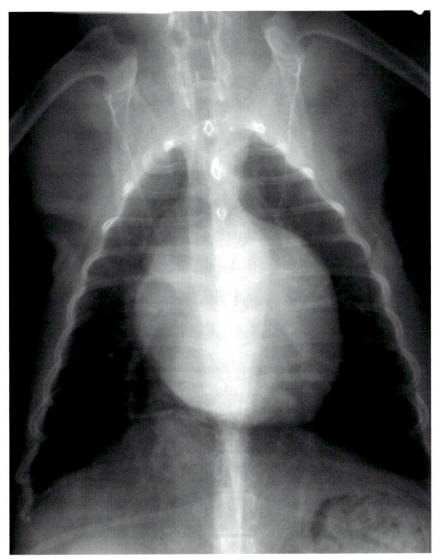

Figure 3-7
Same dog as Figure 3-6. Note enlarged left atrium and auricle.

Causes of Left-Sided Heart Enlargement

✓ Congenital lesions may cause left-sided heart enlargement in neonates younger than than 1 year.

✓ Subvalvular aortic stenosis in dogs (Figures 3-8 and 3-9) or valvular stenosis in cats.

♥ Common and can be very subtle. Often the left atrium is not appreciably enlarged. Because the hypertrophy is concentric, the outside contour of the heart may be minimally enlarged. The disease usually progresses to include eccentric hypertrophy of both the atrium and ventricle, resulting in obvious enlargement of both chambers.

✓ Often occurs in Newfoundlands and other large breed dogs.

✓ Patent ductus arteriosum (PDA) in dogs and cats.

♥ Classic bulge in region of aortic aneurysm (1 to 2 o'clock on VD/DV view). The bulge merges with the contour of the remainder of the descending aorta.

✓ Signs of left atrial and ventricular enlargement are usual.

✓ Enlarged pulmonary arteries and veins are a result of overcirculation.

✋ **Don't miss this disease!** These animals can go into failure at a young age unless detected and treated.

✓ PDA is common in Poodles, Pomeranians, German Shepherds, Collies, and Shelties.

✓ Ventricular septal defect (dogs and cats)

✓ Signs of left atrial and ventricular enlargement are usual with enlarged pulmonary arteries and veins as a result of overcirculation.

✓ Common in Bulldogs.

✓ Most common anomaly in cats.

✓ Mitral valve dysplasia (dogs and cats)

✓ Signs of left atrial and ventricular enlargement are usual.

✓ Often the left atrium is disproportionately enlarged compared with the ventricular enlargement.

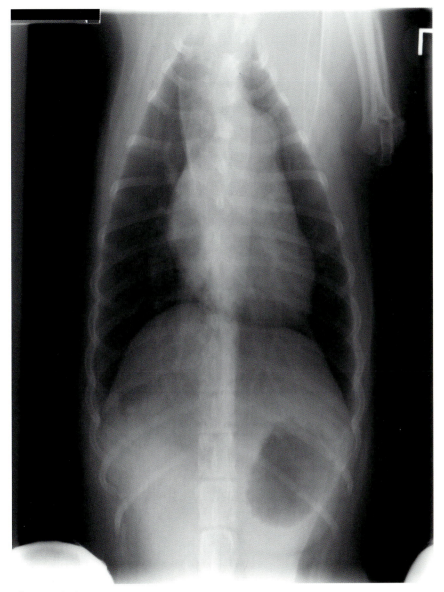

Figure 3-8
A 3 month old female Alaskan Malamute with aortic stenosis. Note increased length (on VD) and height (on lateral view) of heart (subtle) and increased size of aortic arch.

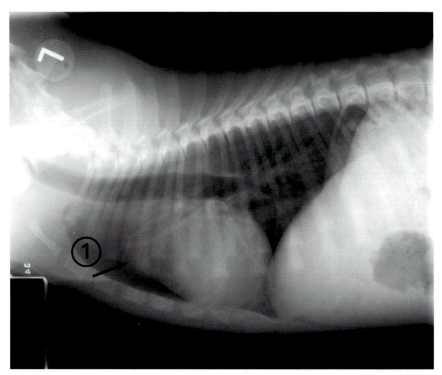

Figure 3-9
Lateral view of Alaskan Malamute in Figure 3-8 showing mild increased height of heart and size of aortic arch (1).

- ✓ Pulmonary venous enlargement indicates pulmonary congestion.
- ✓ Common in German Shepherds, Great Danes, Bull Terriers, Golden Retrievers, Newfoundlands, and Mastiffs.

- ✓ Endocardial cushion defect (cats) (high ventricular septal defect, low atrial septal defect, or both).
  - ✓ Signs of gross left atrial and ventricular enlargement are usual with enlarged pulmonary arteries and veins from over circulation.

- ✓ Early onset of acquired diseases
  - ✓ In older patients, think acquired diseases.
  - ✓ Cardiomyopathies in dogs and cats.

Cats

✓ Hypertrophic cardiomyopathy is the most common cause in cats.

   ♥ Gross left atrial enlargement resulting in valentine-shaped heart on VD/DV. Remember the normal almond shaped heart!

   ♥ Subtle left ventricular enlargement (tall/long heart).

   ✓ Enlarged pulmonary veins (if lungs are congested).

   ✓ Pulmonary edema (if decompensated failure).

✓ Dilated cardiomyopathy (uncommon now).

   ♥ All chambers enlarged—you will see a round heart.

   ♥ Pleural effusion if right-sided heart failure.

   ✓ Enlarged pulmonary veins if lungs congested (compensated left-side heart failure).

   ✓ Pulmonary edema if decompensated left-sided heart failure.

✓ Hyperthyroid cardiomyopathy is a common cause.

   ♥ Normal to subtle left-sided enlargement.

   ✓ Signs of failure uncommon.

   ♥ These patients are sensitive to fluid overload. This easily puts some cats into heart failure.

✓ Systemic hypertension

   ♥ Secondary to renal failure, or idiopathic.

   ✓ Normal to subtle left-sided enlargement.

   ✓ Signs of failure rare.

   ♥ These patients are sensitive to fluid overload. This easily puts some cats into heart failure.

Dogs

✓ Dilated cardiomyopathy (DCM) is a common cause—more in large breeds but seen in breeds as small as Cocker Spaniels.

- ♥ Left and right atrial and ventricular enlargement (round heart).
- ♥ Peritoneal effusion (if right-sided failure) is more common than pleural effusion.
- ✓ Enlarged pulmonary veins (if lungs congested).
- ✓ Pulmonary edema (if decompensated left-sided heart failure).
- ✓ Subclassification of DCM.

✋Primary inotropic disease is common in Doberman Pinschers, but be aware that normal heart size is a distinct possibility for DCM in Dobermans.

- ♥ Can present with signs of left- or right-sided failure with normal heart size.
- ♥ Diagnosis is made by echocardiography.

♥ Primary arrythmias, especially ventricular tachycardia, are common in Boxers.

- ♥ Can present with signs of left- or right-sided failure with normal heart size.
- ✋ As with Dobermans, a normal heart size does not discount the possibility of DCM in a Boxer.
- ♥ Diagnosis often requires ECG.

✓ Valvular disease is more common in dogs than cats.

♥ Mitral valve insufficiency is very common in dogs and rare in cats.

- ♥ Found in small-breed dogs, especially cavalier King Charles Spaniels.
- ✓ Endocardiosis of valve leaflets: valves are affected in the following order of frequency–mitral valve, tricuspid valve, aortic valve, and pulmonic valve.
- ✓ Endocarditis is rare.
- ✓ Usually see signs of left atrial and ventricular enlargement.
- ✓ Pulmonary venous enlargement (pulmonary congestion).

Signs of Right-Sided Heart Enlargement

✓ Cardiomegaly (per verterbral scale system).

✓ Right atrial and ventricular enlargement (per clock face method).

♥ Severe right-sided enlargement can result in generalized cardiomegaly.

✓ Right atrial enlargement

Lateral projection (usually not seen)

Bulging at 9 to 12 o'clock (auricle)

VD/DV projection

Bulging 9 to 12 o'clock

✓ Right ventricular enlargement

Lateral projection

A wide heart

Rounding at 6 to 9 o'clock

♥ Apex of heart elevated off sternum (especially in right lateral view).

🖐 Increased sternal contact of heart is NOT a useful sign.

VD/DV projection

A wide heart

Rounding at 6 to 9 o'clock

Apex shifted further to left

✓ Concurrent abnormalities

✓ Increased width of caudal vena cava. See Vessels section.

♥ Right-sided failure with peritoneal effusion (in dogs more commonly than cats), and pleural effusion (in cats more commonly than dogs).

Causes of Right-Sided Enlargement

✓ Congenital

✓ Tricuspid valve dysplasia (common in dogs, uncommon in cats) (Figure 3-10)

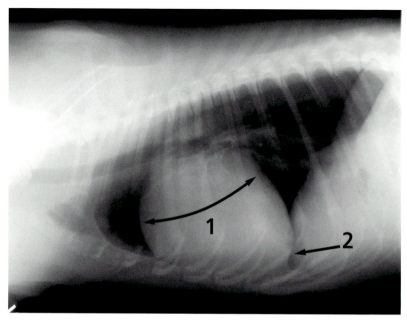

Figure 3-10
An 8 month old male neutered Labrador Retriever with tricuspid valve insufficiency. Note the increased width of the heart (1) and elevation of heart (2).

- ✓ Usually see signs of right atrial and ventricular enlargement (rounded heart shape).
- ✓ Signs of right heart failure (see above).
- ✓ Found in Labrador Retrievers, Weimaraners, German Shepherds, Old English Sheepdogs.
- ✓ Pulmonic valve stenosis in both dogs and cats
  - ✓ Found in Bulldogs, Bassett Hounds, Beagles, Boykin Spaniels, Schnauzers, Terriers, and Boxers.
  - ♥ Can be very subtle.
  - ✓ Often the heart is not appreciably enlarged. Because the hypertrophy is concentric, the outside contour may not be enlarged.
  - ♥ Look for a bump in 1 to 2 o'clock position.
  - ✓ Pulmonary vessels will appear normal or small.
- ✓ Acquired diseases—happens in dogs more than in cats.

- ✓ Pulmonary hypertension
  - ✓ Uncommon
  - ✓ Often the heart is not appreciably enlarged. Because the hypertrophy is concentric, the outside contour may not be enlarged.
  - ♥ Look for a bump in 1 to 2 o'clock position.
  - ✓ Pulmonary arteries are enlarged and undulating, and pulmonary veins appear normal or small.
  - ✓ Causes of pulmonary hypertension
    - ✓ Heartworm disease (Figures 3-11 and 3-12).
      - ✓ Appears more often in dogs more than cats.
      - ✓ Additional pulmonary lesions can include granulmas, edema, and pneumonia.
    - ✓ Idiopathic
    - ✓ Primary pulmonary fibrosis can cause right-sided enlargement in West Highland White Terriers.
    - ✓ Chronic obstructive pulmonary disease.
    - ✓ Chronic left heart failure.

Signs of Generalized Cardiomegaly

- ✓ Cardiomegaly (per verterbral scale system)
- ✓ Left- and right-sided cardiomegaly (per clockface system).
- ✓ Round heart on lateral and VD/DV projections.
- ✓ Concurrent abnormalities: right-sided signs are present more often than left-sided signs.

Causes of Generalized Cardiomegaly

- ✓ Congenital in dogs and cats.
- ✓ Severe right more often than left-sided anomalies.
- ✓ Tricuspid valve dysplasia more often than mitral valve dysplasia.

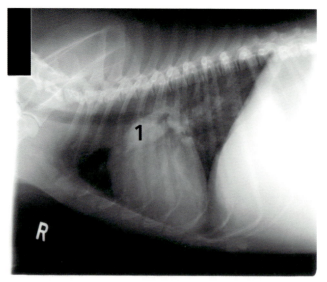

Figure 3-11
An 8 year old female spayed Springer Spaniel with pulmonary hypertension caused by infestation with heartworms showing the increased width of the cranial lobar artery (1).

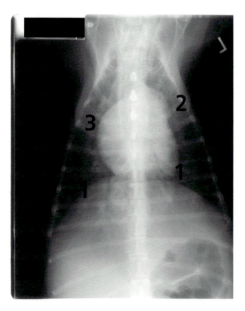

Figure 3-12
Same patient as Figure 3-11. In addition to the increased width of the cranial lobar arteries (1), note the size of main pulmonary trunk (2), and the slight right atrial enlargement (3).

♥ Pericardial peritoneal diaphragmatic hernia causes apparent cardiomegaly in cats more than in dogs (see Diaphragm section).

✔ It mimics a round heart, usually is incidental in cats, and causes clinical signs if there is entrapment of viscera.

✔ Acquired causes

✔ Difficult to differentiate causes on radiographs.

✔ Need echocardiography to determine underlying cause.

✔ Cardiomyopathy (Figures 3-13, 3-14, and 3-15)

✔ DCM in dogs. Large breeds are predisposed, but so are Cocker Spaniels.

✔ HCM or DCM in cats (Figures 3-16 and 3-17).

✔ Bilateral atrioventricular valvular insufficiency (mitral and tricuspid valves in dogs (small breed predisposition).

✔ Pericardial effusion in dogs. Large breeds are predisposed (Figure 3-18).

✔ Mimics a round heart.

(*continued on page 60*)

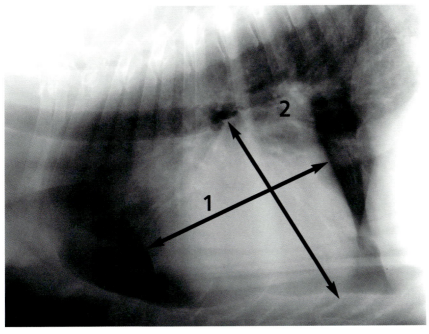

Figure 3-13
An 8 year old male Mastiff with dilated cardiomyopathy. Note generalized (1) cardiomegaly (12.5 vertebrae) including left atrial enlargement (2).

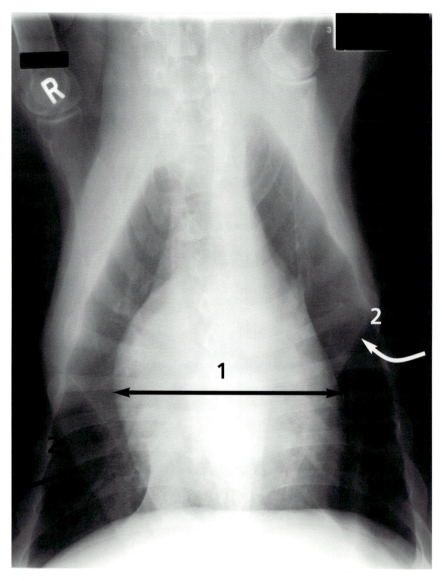

Figure 3-14
Same patient as Figure 3-13. In addition to generalized cardiomegaly
(1), skin folds mimic pleural effusion or pneumothorax (2).

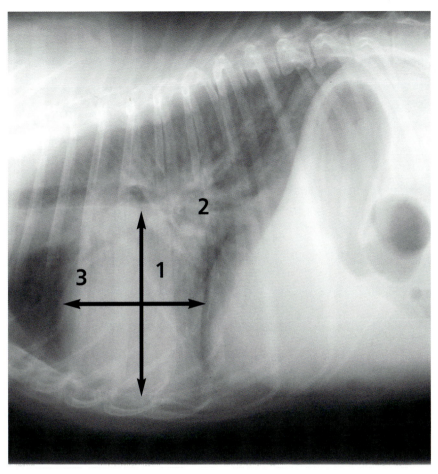

Figure 3-15
A 9 year old male neutered Doberman with cardiomyopathy. The heart size is normal (1) based on vertebral scale method. The left atrial (2) and pulmonary venous (3) enlargement seen here are excellent indicators of this disease in the face of normal cardiac size.

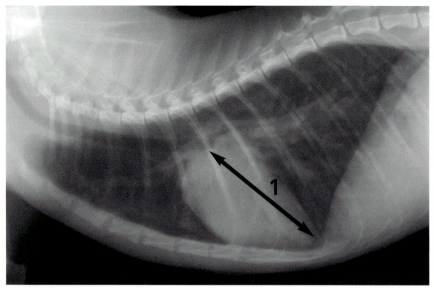

Figure 3-16
A 2 year old male neutered domestic short-hair cat with hypertrophic cardiomyopathy showing mild increased height of the heart (1).

(continued from page 57)

✓ Commonly caused by heart base neoplasia, especially hemangiosarcoma.

Common Causes of Heart Disease with Normal Appearing Heart

✓ ECG abnormality

✓ Pulmonary hypertension

✓ Aortic or pulmonic stenosis

✓ Doberman or Boxer DCM

✓ Fluid overload in cat (or, less often dog).

✓ Any mild valvular insufficiency or congenital anomaly

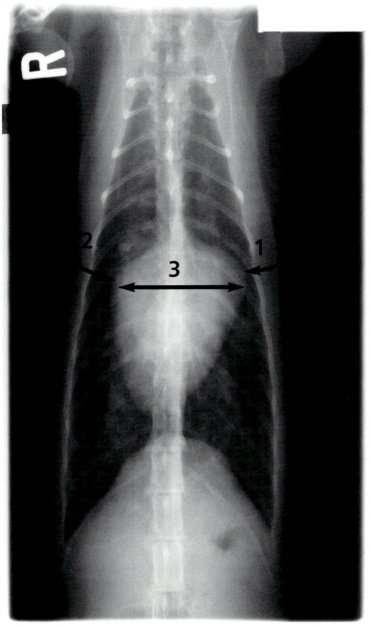

Figure 3-17
In the same cat as Figure 3-16, note the increased size of
the left auricle (1) and right atrium (2). The heart measured
4.5 vertebrae on the vertebral heart scale system (3).

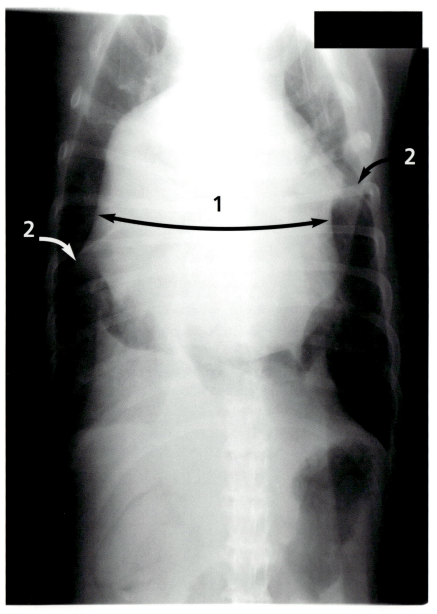

Figure 3-18
A 10 year old male neutered Golden Retriever with pericardial effusion.
Note generalized cardiomegaly (1) and pleural effusion (2).

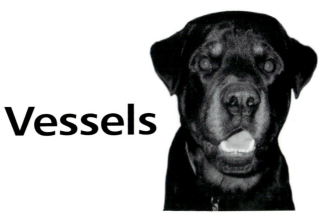

Vessels

Intrathoracic Vasculature

Vessels are often overlooked by the inexperienced. There are three groups of vessels in the chest: aorta, the caudal vena cava, and the pulmonary vessels, arteries, and veins. Each of these should be examined.

♥ Failure to examine the pulmonary vessels is common but is a major mistake.

Intrathoracic Aorta

✓ Is rarely the site of detectable disease.

✓ On lateral projection, an undulation of the aorta is seen. This a common incidental feature in older cats.

♥ The undulation usually does not equate to increased pressure in the aorta.

✓ Systemic hypertension or hypotension results in no detectable size change.

✓ VD/DV view

✓ The aorta is visible to left of midline until it enters diaphragm.

♥ A bump in the cranial portion (1 to 2 o'clock position) is classic for patent ductus arteriosus.

Caudal Vena Cava

✓ Is usually seen on lateral and DV/VD projection in caudal, ventral, and right thorax views.

✓ Its variable size may not be related to the clinical status of the patient.

♥ The upper limit of normal for caudal vena cava diameter on a left lateral projection is 1.3 times the width of the descending aorta and 1.5 times the length of a mid-thoracic vertebra.

✓ Often appears subjectively small in cases of hypovolemia, shock, or dehydration.

Pulmonary Vessels

♥ Are often overlooked portions of the radiograph.

♥ Are an essential feature to tie together heart and lung changes.

✓ Pulmonary veins are "ventral and central" (see following).

General Principles

Lateral projections
- ✓ Limit your evaluation to the cranial lobar vessels.
- ✓ The pair of vessels we see best are the ones in the non dependent lung
- ✓ On the left lateral view, the vessels we see are the right cranial lobar vessels. The pair of vessels in the nondependent lung is more ventral and is magnified to appear larger than the pair in the dependent lung.
- ✓ Notice that arteries are dorsal to the veins.

Normal size relationships

Dog
- ✓ Measured where the vessels cross the 4th rib.
- ✓ The artery and the vein should be the same size.
- 🖐 Normal upper limit: Diameter of the proximal 1/3 of the 4th rib.
- 🖐 Normal lower limit:1/2 diameter of the proximal 1/3 of the 4th rib.
- ♥ Don't compare the vessels to the distal part of the 4th rib (Figures 4-1 and 4-2).

Cat
- 🖐 Many cats have a more caudal-positioned heart than dogs.
- 🖐 Measured where the vessels cross the cranial heart border.
- ✓ The artery and vein should be the same size.
- 🖐 Upper limit of normal is the diameter of the proximal 1/3 of the 4th or 5th rib.
- 🖐 Lower limit of normal is half the diameter of the proximal 1/3 of the 4th or 5th rib.
- ♥ Don't compare the vessels to the distal part of the ribs (Figure 4-3).

VD/DV projection
- ✓ Limit your evaluation to the caudal lobar vessels.
- ✓ Both the left and right caudal lobar pair of vessels are visible.

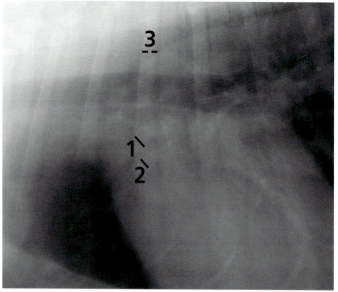

Figure 4-1
Normal 2 year old female spayed Labrador Retriever. Close up of cranial lobar vessels on lateral view. Note that pulmonary artery (1) and vein (2) are narrower than the width of the proximal 1/3 of 4th rib (3) .

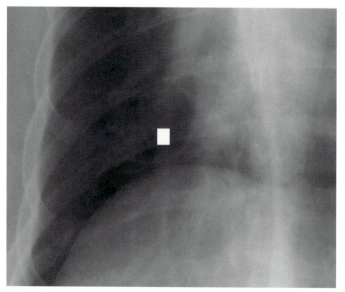

Figure 4-2
Note that the pulmonary artery is narrower than the width of the 9th rib resulting in a rectangle which is longer than wide.

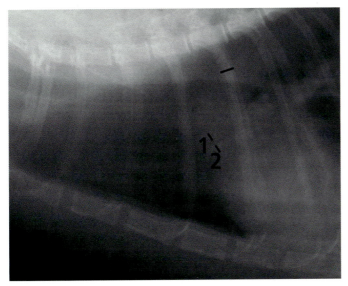

Figure 4-3
Lateral view of 5 year old domestic short-haired cat. Close-up of cranial thorax showing width of pulmonary artery (1) and vein (2) at level of cranial heart relative to width of proximal.

✓ The vessels are better appreciated on the DV view than on the VD view.

✓ Arteries are lateral to the veins

✓ Normal size relationships

Dog

✓ Measured where the vessels cross the 9th rib.

✓ The artery and the vein should be the same size.

✋ Where the vessels cross the rib image, that intersection is a rectangle. If the vessel is wider than the rib, the rectangle will be wider than tall, or abnormal. If the rectangle is taller than wide, (see Figure 4-2) then the vessel is within normal limits of size.

✋ Upper limit of normal is the diameter of the 9th rib where they cross.

✋ Lower limit of normal is half the diameter of the 9th rib where they cross.

Cat

✋ Many cats have a more caudal-positioned heart than dogs.

✋ Measured where the vessels cross 10th rib.

✓ Artery should be the same size as the vein.

🖐 Diameter of the 10th rib where vessels cross.

🖐 1/2 diameter of the 10th rib where vessels cross.

Radiologic Signs of Vascular Disease

There are only four combinations of radiographic abnormalities.

🖐 Any discrepancy between artery and vein is abnormal; the larger vessel is abnormal.

1. Both the arteries and veins are enlarged (Figures 4-4 and 4-5).

♥ Overcirculation

✓ In a young animal, consider a left-to-right shunting a cardiac anomaly.

✓ Patent ductus arteriosus

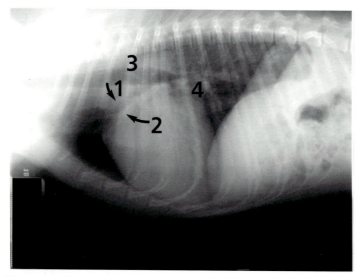

Figure 4-4
Patent ductus arteriosus in a 2 year old female Cocker Spaniel. Pulmonary overcirculation is evidenced by enlarged pulmonary arteries (1) and veins (2) compared to the proximal rib (3). The left atrium is also enlarged (4).

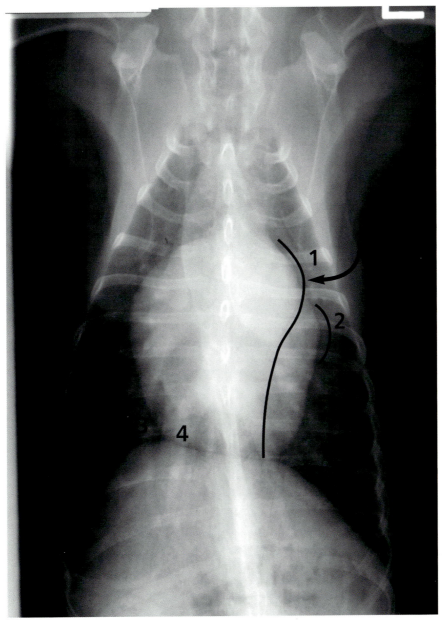

Figure 4-5
The same Cocker Spaniel as in Figure 4-4. Note the increased size of the aorta (traced line) at the site of the aneurysm (1), left auricle (2). Pulmonary overcirculation as evidenced by enlarged pulmonary arteries (3) and veins (4).

✓ Ventricular septal defect

✓ Atrial septal defect

♥ Severe chronic left-sided heart failure (see below under big veins)

2. Both the arteries and veins are small (Figure 4-6).

♥ Hypovolemia, shock, and dehydration are common secondary to noncardiac disease.

✓ In a young animal, consider a right-to-left shunting cardiac anomaly (tetralogy of Fallot, reverse patent ductus arteriosus).

✓ Severe pulmonic stenosis

3. Arteries are enlarged, but the veins are normal (see Figures 3-11 and 3-12).

♥ Arteries commonly undulate, become tortuous in appearance.

✓ Pulmonary hypertension

✓ Heartworm disease: In cats, the artery is less than 4 mm at the level of the 9th rib on VD view.

✓ Chronic pulmonary thromboembolic disease.

✓ Chronic obstructive pulmonary disease (COPD).

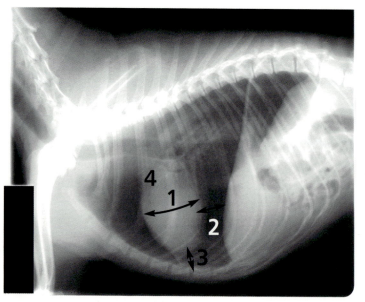

Figure 4-6
This is a 5 year old male neutered Sheltie in shock after being hit by a car. The heart size is small (1) with increased distance between it and the diaphragm (2), the sternum (3), and the small pulmonary arteries and veins (4).

✓ Idiopathic

4. Veins are enlarged but the arteries are normal (Figure 4-7).

   ✓ Most common abnormality in older patients with heart disease.

   ♥ Pulmonary congestion

      ♥ Cardiomyopathy in cats and dogs

      ♥ Mitral valve insufficiency (dogs)

      ♥ Iatrogenic fluid overload occurs more often in cats than in dogs.

   ♥ An important sign of left-sided heart failure.

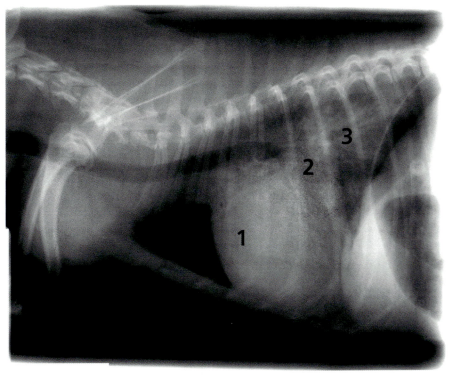

Figure 4-7
A 4 year old female spayed Chihuahua. Pulmonary venous congestion (1), left atrial enlargement (2), and pulmonary edema (3) are seen.

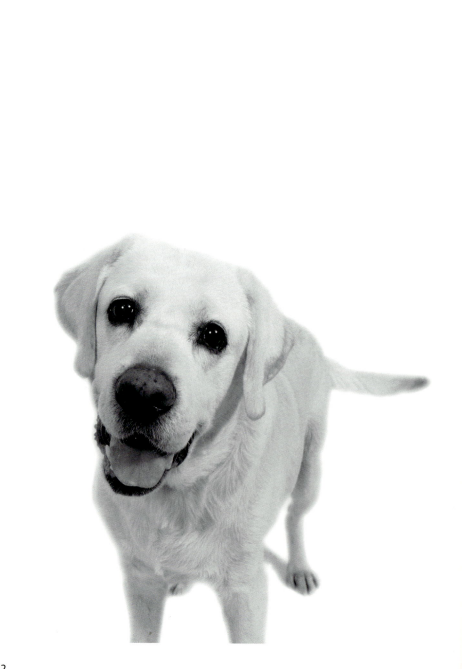

Section 5

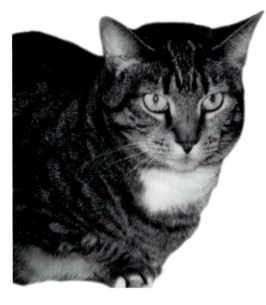

Lungs

The lungs are one of the most important subjects of radiographic interpretation. The main question when viewing radiographs is "Are the lungs too opaque or too lucent?" If they are too opaque, see the following discussion on the pattern system. If they are too lucent, read the discussion at the end of this chapter. The pattern approach to interpreting lung lesions can simplify your life since it organizes what you are seeing. Mixed patterns are common, but will not be discussed here. If you are faced with one, try to identify the most severe one—alveolar or nodular. For a review of common normal variants, see the section on radiographic anatomy.

Causes of Increased Lung Opacity: The Pattern Approach

The pattern seen on images can help determine the causes of lung opacity. Common variations in patterns are:

♥ On expiration, a mild interstitial pattern (Figures 5-1 and 5-2).

♥ If the film is underexposed, a mild interstitial pattern may be seen.

♥ In geriatric patients, mild bronchial and interstitial patterns are common.

♥ A mild interstitial pattern is seen in obesity.

✓ Heterotopic bone mimic nodules in Collies.

✓ Nipples, ticks, dirt, and costochondral junctions mimic pulmonary nodules.

♥ The patterns of increased pulmonary opacity are:
  ♥ Alveolar
  ✓ Bronchial
  ✓ Vascular
  ♥ Nodular interstitial
  ✓ Unstructured interstitial

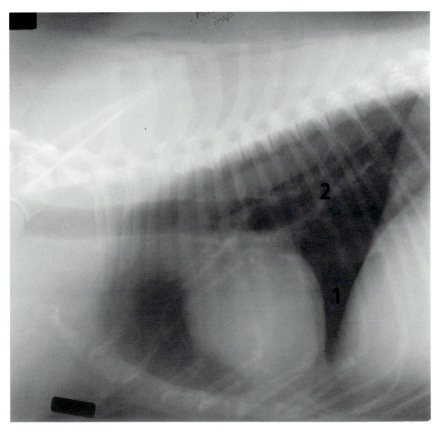

Figure 5-1

On inspiration in this 7 year old Golden Retriever, there is a greater distance between the heart and diaphragm (1) resulting in a well-defined triangle of lucent lung ventral to the caudal vena cava, caudal to the heart and cranial to the diaphragm. The lungs are more lucent (2) than in Figure 5-2.

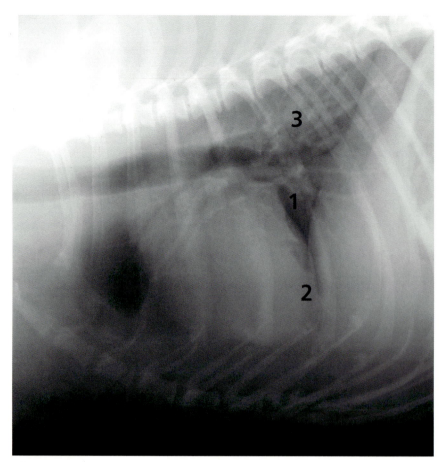

Figure 5-2

On expiration in the same animal, the caudal ventral triangle of lung is much smaller (1). There is overlap of the heart and diaphragm (2), and the lungs appear more opaque (3).

Alveolar Patterns

Features of alveolar patterns include:

♥ A silhouette sign which is the inability to see margins of the heart, vessels, and diaphragm. The silhouette sign is the most important and dependable feature of the alveolar pattern.

✓ Air bronchogram, a variation of silhouette sign.

Air can be seen in the bronchial lumen surrounded by opaque lung. It has been described as a black tree branching in a snow storm.

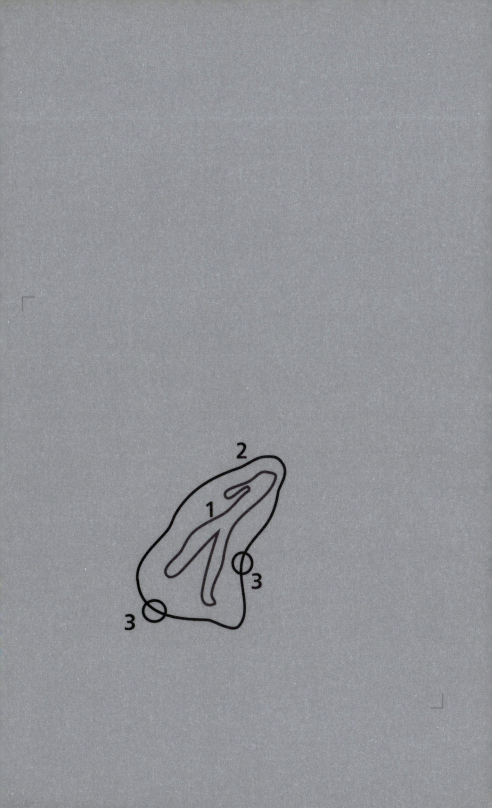

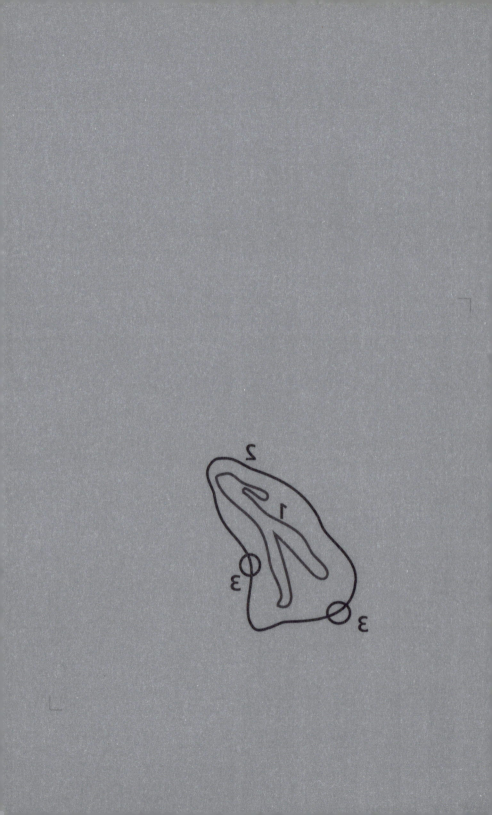

✓ Lobar sign: the disease margins are limited precisely by the lung lobe margin and the disease seems to completely fill one lobe.

✓ Distribution: explanation of terms

    ✓ Lobar: completely filled lobe, no aerated alveoli.

    ✓ Patchy nonconsolidating: hazy margins, small parts of more than one lobe.

    ✓ Regional: distinct margins, not involving the entire lobe, possibly involving more than one lobe.

The following describes typical alveolar findings, their possible causes, and testing options.

✓ Pus (bronchopneumonia) (Figures 5-3 and 5-4)

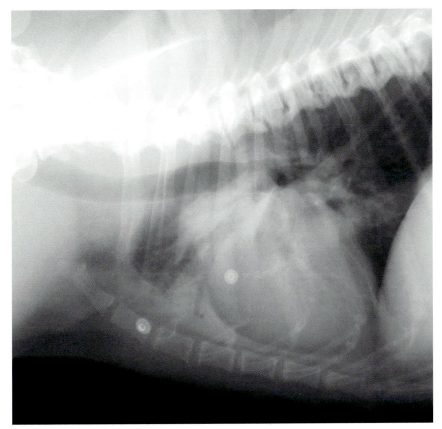

Figure 5-3

Air bronchogram in pneumonia (1). Lobar sign (2) at the edge of the consolidated lung. ECG leads (3).

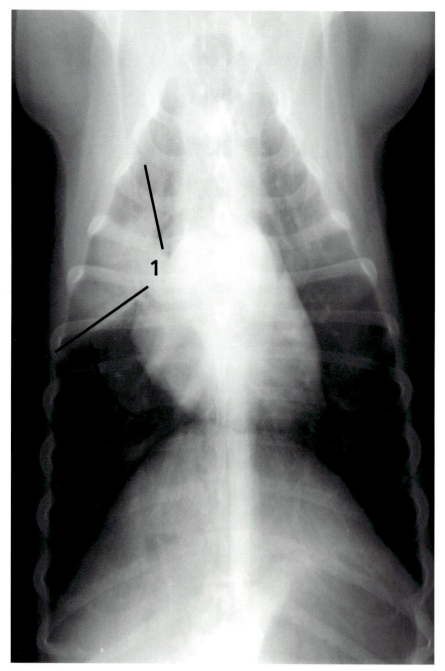

Figure 5-4
Bronchogram of pneumonia. Note lobar sign (arrow) and silhouetting with the heart margin in the region where the pneumonia touches the heart (1).

- ✔ Neutrophilic, eosinophilic, or granulocytic infiltration
- ✔ Usually a cranial/middle ventral distribution
- ✔ Distribution: lobar, nonconsolidating, or widespread regional
- ✋ Diffuse only after death
- ✔ Blood
  - ✔ Hemorrhage, contusions, torsion, thromboembolism
  - ✔ Site of focal trauma–look for rib fractures
  - ✔ Distribution: free blood will eventually fall to a ventral or dependent location
- ✔ Cells (neoplasia)
  - ✔ Lymphoma (in dogs)
  - ✔ Primary lung neoplasia (in cats)
  - ✔ Atypical metastasis
  - ✔ Distribution: lobar to patchy nonconsolidating
- ✔ Water (edema)
  - ♥ Secondary to left-sided heart failure (Figures 5-5 and 5-6)
    - ✔ Distribution
      - ♥ Dogs: hilar nonconsolidating
      - ✋ Cats: widespread patchy or hilar nonconsolidating
  - ♥ Noncardiogenic conditions (neurogenic or vasculitis)
    - ✔ Secondary to seizures, neck, or head trauma
    - ✔ Vascular permeability diseases, such as DIC and pancreatitis
    - ✔ Distribution: bilateral regional (caudodorsal)
- ✔ Empty lung
  - ✔ Atelectasis, lung collapse, torsion
  - ✔ Reduced volume compared to normal
  - ✔ Acute: evidence of mediastinal shift (see Mediastinum)
  - ✔ Distribution: lobar or regional
- ✔ Testing options
  - ✔ Direct
    - ✔ Rule out heart failure through echocardiography or electrocardiography.

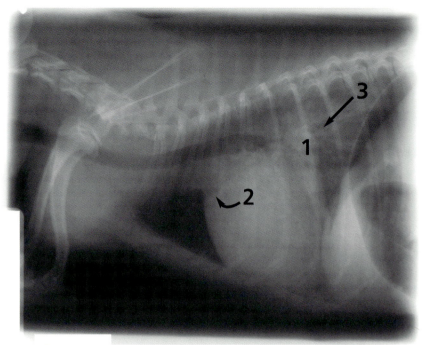

Figure 5-5
Secondary pulmonary edema associated with uncompensated left-sided heart failure due to mitral valve insufficiency in a 4 year old female spayed Chihuahua. Note the left atrial enlargement (1), pulmonary venous congestion (2), and perihilar increased pulmonary opacity in an interstitial and alveolar pattern (3) representing edema.

- ✓ Elicit history of seizures and perform a neurologic examination.
- ✓ Tracheal wash, bronchial-alveolar lavage (BAL)
- ✓ Ultrasound-guided aspirate/biopsy
✓ Indirect
  - ✓ Complete blood count
  - ✓ Coagulation panel
  - ✓ Assess response to therapy (diuretics, antibiotics).

🖑 In cats, the differential diagnosis for patchy nonconsolidating alveolar disease (Figures 5-7 and 5-8) includes:
  - 🖑 Left-sided heart failure (edema).
  - 🖑 Primary lung neoplasia (with or without mineralization).
  - 🖑 Mycoplasma pneumonia (with or without mineralization).

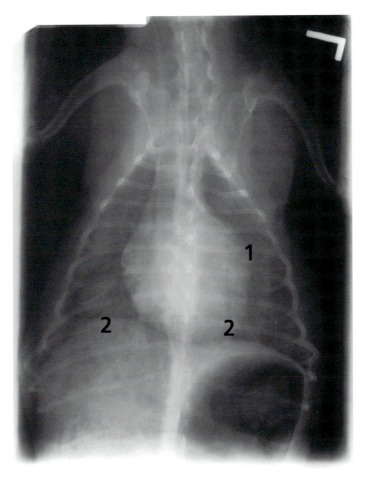

Figure 5-6
In the same patient as Figure 5-5, you can see the enlarged left auricle
(1) and bilateral pulmonary edema (2).

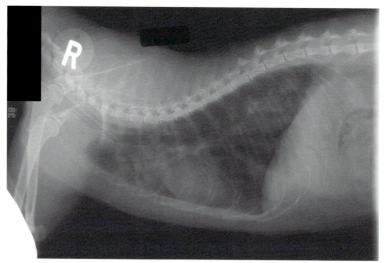

Figure 5-7
Lateral view of 10 year old female domestic short haired cat with
pulmonary adenocarcinoma. Note patchy alveolar pattern in all lung fields.

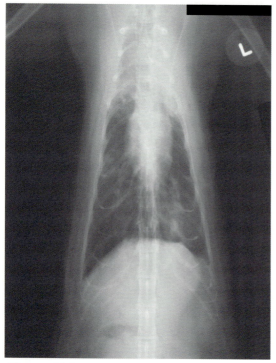

Figure 5-8
Ventral dorsal view of the same cat (Figure 5-7), note patchy alveolar
pattern in both lungs.

Bronchial Patterns

✓ The following section describes typical bronchial findings, their possible causes, and testing options (Figures 5-9, 5-10, 5-11, and 5-12).

✓ Thickened bronchi

   ✓ Infiltration with inflammatory cells/edema

   ♥ Bronchitis

      🖐 In dogs, bacterial bronchitis is more common than allergic (eosinophilic).

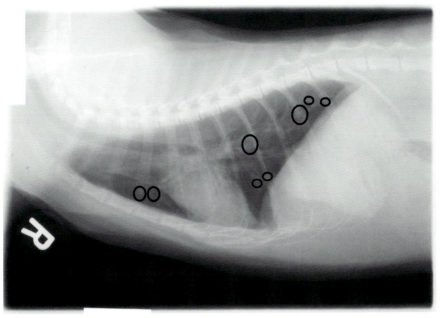

Figure 5-9
Lateral view of 3 year old domestic short-haired cat with chronic bronchitis. Note the thickened bronchi (circles).

   🖐 In cats, allergic bronchitis is more common than bacterial (*Mycoplasma* species)

✓ Opaque (normal-thickness) bronchi

   ✓ Normal in geriatric patients

   ✓ Residual mineralization secondary to chronic (may or may not be active) bronchitis.

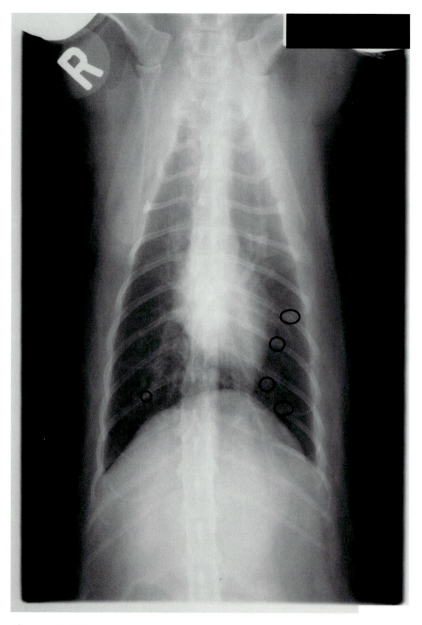

Figure 5-10
Ventral dorsal view of same cat as in Figure 5-9. Note the thickened bronchi (circles).

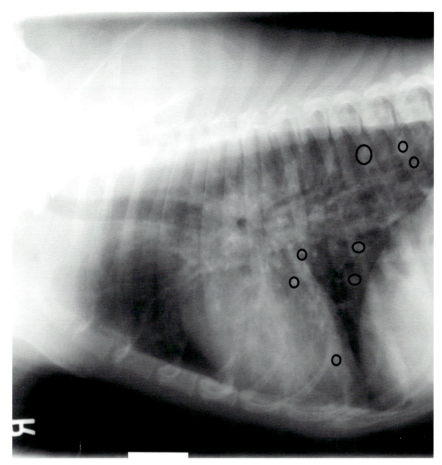

Figure 5-11
Lateral view of 4 year old female German short haired pointer with
eosinophilic bronchitis. Note thickened bronchial walls (circles).

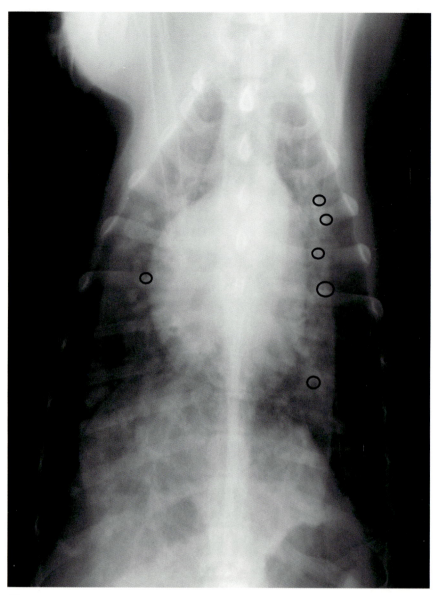

Figure 5-12
Same dog as in Figure 5-11. Note thickened bronchial walls (circles).

- ✓ Widened bronchi
  - ✓ Bronchiectasis
    - ✓ Secondary to chronic bronchopneumonia (see the discussion of pus under alveolar patterns)
    - ✓ Congenital
    - ✓ Predisposes to bronchopneumonia
- ✓ Testing
  - ✓ Direct
    - ✓ Tracheal wash (culture and cytology), BAL
  - ✓ Indirect
    - ✓ Complete blood count
    - ✓ Measurement of response to therapy (antibiotics, corticosteroids)

Vascular Patterns
- ✓ Enlarged vessels are the sole cause of increased opacity (see Heart)

Nodular Interstitial
- ✓ Soft tissue opacity
  - ♥ Normal variations
    - ✓ Mineralized costochondral junctions
    - ✓ Nipples, ticks, dirt on skin
  - ✓ End-on pulmonary arteries or veins
  - ✓ Round, varying-sized masses:
    - ✓ Miliary = size of a millet seed (see Figure 5-8).
    - ✓ Other masses can be described in terms of vegetable or fruit sizes such as pea, grape, orange, etc.
    - 🖐 Some masses may mimic the appearance of a second heart!
    - ✓ No silhouette sign
  - ✓ Causes
    - ✓ Metastatic neoplasia (Figure 5-13)
    - ✓ Primary neoplasia (Figure 5-14), often mixed with air or mineralized foci
    - ✓ Mycotic pneumonia
    - ✓ Granuloma

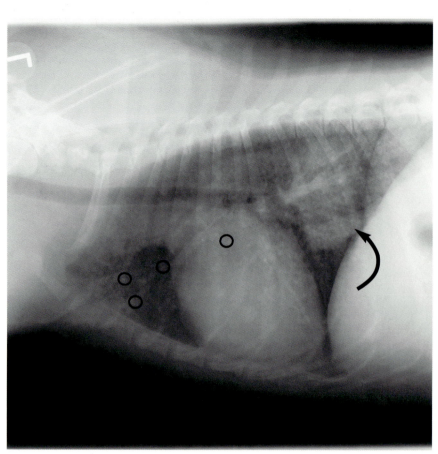

Figure 5-13
Lateral view of 8 year old female spayed Golden Retriever with metastatic osteosarcoma. The metastatic nodules vary in size from miliary (circles) to very large (arrow).

  ✔ Abscess
  ✔ Hematoma, hematocele
 ♥ Normal variations (see previous chapters)
  ✔ Mineralized costochondral junctions
  ✔ Dirt on the skin
  ✔ Heterotopic bone in Collies and other breeds
  ✔ Bronchial abnormalities (see preceding discussion)
 ✔ Discrete mineralization focus
  ✔ Primary lung neoplasia (cats and dogs)

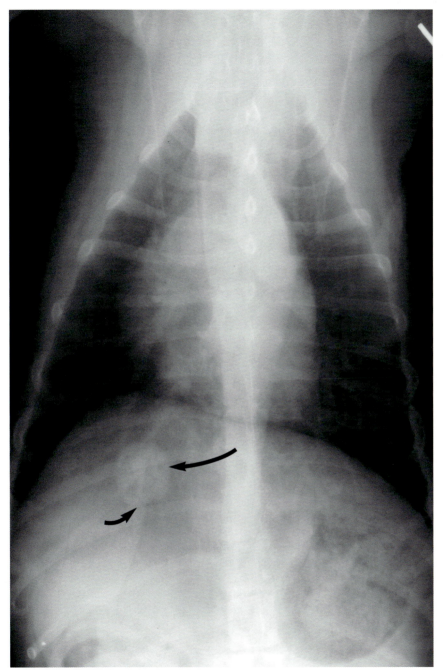

Figure 5-14
Primary lung neoplasia in right caudal lung lobe (arrows). Note cavitated appearance: soft tissue and air opacity make a mixed opacity mass.

- ✓ Chronic bronchopneumonia (cats with *Mycoplasma* infection)
- ✓ Hilar lymph node (mycotic, neoplasia, aspirated barium)
- ✓ Reticular/linear pattern
  - ✓ Hypercalcemia
  - ✓ Hypercortisolism (caused by endogenous or exogenous corticosteroids)
  - ✓ Uremia

Unstructured Interstitial

🖐 Overdiagnosed as an abnormal pattern

🖐 Common as a normal variant under the following conditions:

- ♥ Expiration
- ♥ Underexposure
- ♥ Geriatric patients
- ♥ Obesity

🖐 Requires a high degree of skill to differentiate normal variants from true disease.

- ✓ Causes
  - ♥ Lymphoma (diffuse) (Figure 5-15)
  - ♥ Nonalveolarized regional edema (edema that is forming or resolving)
    - ✓ Left-sided heart failure (regional; see preceding discussion)
    - ✓ Vasculitis (regional to diffuse; see preceding discussion)
    - ✓ Atypical allergic/infectious pneumonitis (regional to diffuse)
- ✓ Testing
  - ♥ Make sure the pattern is not a normal variation.
    - ✓ Complete inspiration?
    - ✓ Good technique?
    - ✓ More opaque than to be expected in other old or obese dogs?
  - ♥ Test for lymphoma!

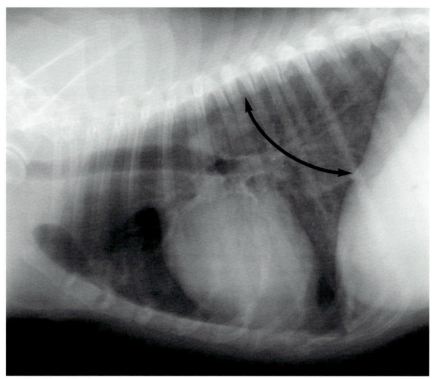

Figure 5-15
Pulmonary lymphoma shows a diffuse unstructured interstitial pattern.
A hazy indistinct increased opacity (arrow) appears with no silhouetting
or thickened bronchi.

Causes of Decreased Opacity

Pneumothorax is discussed in the Pleura chapter.

✓ Diffuse

  ✓ Normal variation

    ✓ Hyperinflation (Figure 5-16) which can result in excited, scared, or hyperthyroid cats.

    ✓ Emaciation

    ✓ Overexposure

    ✓ Overdeveloping of film

  ✓ Pathologic causes

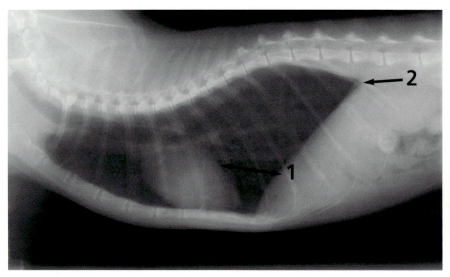

Figure 5-16
Radiograph showing increased lung lucency with increased distance between heart and diaphragm (1) and displaced caudal margin of the lung (2).

✓ Hyperinflation
  ✓ Lower airway disease (that is, air trapping)
    ♥ "Asthmatic" cats
    ✓ Foreign body
  ✓ Some upper airway diseases (most of which cause hypoinflation)
✓ Emphysema
  ✓ Secondary to chronic obstructive pulmonary disease
  ✓ Congenital
✓ Bronchiectasis (see preceding discussion)

Radiographic findings
✓ Increased distance between heart and diaphragm (Figure 5-17)
✓ Tentings of attachment of diaphragm to body wall
✓ Diaphragm extends caudal to T12

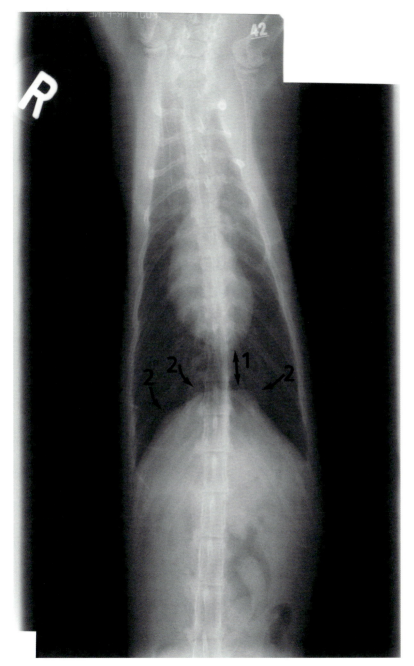

Figure 5-17
In the same patient as Figure 5-11, the increased distance between heart and diaphragm is apparent (1) as is the tenting of the diaphragm due to hyperinflation (2).

- ✓ Regional
  - ✓ Usually a normal variation, especially when it is ventral to the heart on lateral projections and is secondary to hyperinflation
  - ✓ Mimics pneumothorax
- ✓ Focal
  - ✓ Bulla (bleb, cyst, pneumatocele) (Figure 5-18)
    - ✓ Clinically relevant because of association with pneumothorax
    - ✓ Traumatic pneumothorax (air-filled or partially blood-filled)
    - ✓ Congenital (primary pneumothorax)
    - ✓ For increased detectability take expiratory radiographs.
    - ♥ Potential catastrophic pneumothorax if it bursts!
- ♥ The peracute severe dypsneic patient:
  - Consider therapy before imaging
    - ✓ Violation of sacrosanct radiology tenant?
    - ✓ Realistic approach to keeping your patients alive
- ♥ The Big Four
  - ✓ Not the only diseases that cause peracute dyspnea (pneumonia, cancer, etc.). Other diseases we can not reverse. These diseases should be treated within minutes. Empirical therapy: oxygen, low stress environment
  - ✓ These are the diseases that require rapid specific therapy to save a patient's life (Table 5-1).

Table 5-1 Diseases Requiring Fast Specific Therapy

Disease	Direct Therapy
♥ Cardiogenic pulmonary edema	Diuretics
♥ Feline acute asthma complex	Corticosteroids/bronchodilators
♥ Massive pleural effusion	Thoracocentesis
♥ Massive pneumothorax	Thoracocentesis

- ♥ Radiological presentation of cats with bronchial disease (feline asthma complex)
  - ♥ Acute
    - ♥ Hyperinflated or normal

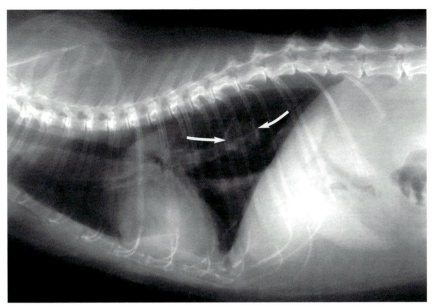

Figure 5-18
Lateral view of 13 year old male neutered domestic short haired cat with pulmonary bulla (arrows).

- ✓ +/- Bronchial pattern
- ✓ +/- Right middle lobe collapse
- ✓ Chronic
  - ✓ Bronchial pattern
  - ✓ Right middle lobe collapse common
  - ✓ Lobar bronchopneumonia common
  - ✓ Normal to hypo-inflated thorax
- ✓ Acute exacerbation of chronic disease
  - ✓ Bronchial pattern
  - ✓ Hyperinflation

Summary
- ✓ Hyperinflated, hypoinflated or normal
- ✓ Bronchial pattern or normal
- ✓ Bronchopneumonia, lung collapse, or normal
- 🖐Note: a normal appearing chest in a dyspneic cat is very reasonable in a cat with feline asthma complex.

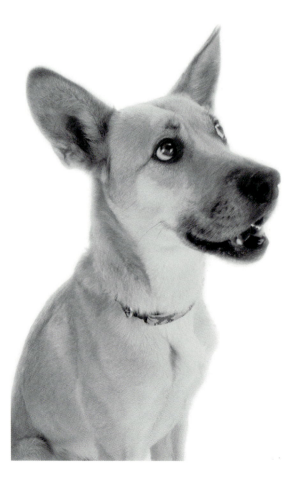

Section 6

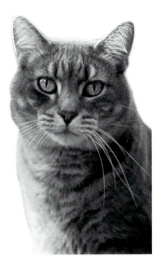

Pleural Space Disease

Two of the peracute diseases that frequently cause death are pleural diseases: pneumothorax and pleural effusion (see Lungs). Normal variations may lead you to misdiagnose these two diseases.

Pneumothorax

♥ The following are normal conditions or other situations that can mimic pneumothorax in cats or dogs:

✔ On ventro-dorsal (VD)/dorsal-ventro (DV) projection, skin folds give the impression of a lucent area lateral to the folds (see Figure 3-14).

♥ On lateral projections, air-filled lung between the cardiac apex and sternum may be seen in the following conditions or types of patients:

✔ Hyperinflation

✔ Emaciation

✔ Very deep- and narrow-chested dog breeds

✔ Patients with microcardia (hypovolemia, right-to-left shunting)

✔ Dogs in left lateral recumbency

✔ Any cause of mediastinal shift (see Diaphragm).

♥ Be fastidious about examining the lucent areas of each radiograph.

✔ Use a bright light to look for vessels or bronchi.

✔ Structures in the lucent areas indicate the lung, not free air.

Physiology of Free Air and Radiographic Views

When obtaining and viewing radiographs for possible pneumothorax, keep in mind that gas rises.

✔ The DV view is the best view for pneumothorax detection because gas should be placed in the widest part of the chest. This view also allows detection of asymmetrical pneumothorax.

✔ Lateral projection is the view most sensitive for a small pneumothorax and can show separation of the lung from the diaphragm or ribs (Figure 6-1).

✓ When the lung is not air-filled, the heart can fall to a more dependent location.

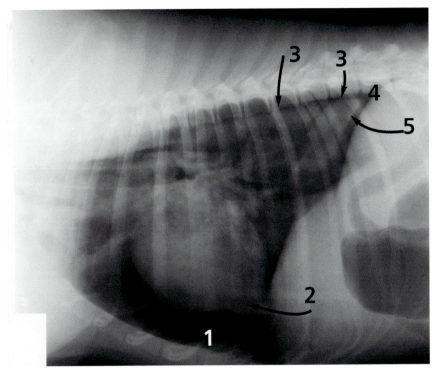

Figure 6-1

Pneumothorax. This dog was hit by a car. Note the increased lucency and distance ventral to the heart representing free pleural air (1), dorsal displacement of the heart away from the sternum (2), ventral displacement of the lungs away from the dorsal-most arch of the ribs (3), increased lucency with no vessels or bronchi in the caudodorsal-most thorax (4), and cranial displacement of the lung margin away from the diaphragm (5).

Roentgen Signs

✓ Lateral projection

    ✓ Shows "elevation" of heart away from sternum.

    ✓ On this view, pneumothorax is the only instance in which an abnormality outside the lung is less opaque than structures in the normal lung. As a result, you'll see an opaque lung border that is summated on or ventral to spine and is cranial to the diaphragm (Figure 6-1).

✓ DV/VD projection

    ✓ On this view, you'll also see an opaque lung border and retraction of lung borders away from the ribs.

✓ Both views

    ✓ Partial collapse: mild to moderate interstitial pattern

    ✓ Complete lobe or lung collapse: alveolar pattern

    ♥ Contusion or hemorrhage: focal patchy increased interstitial or alveolar pattern

Underlying Causes

♥ Trauma

    ✓ Rib fractures

    ✓ Pulmonary contusions

    ✓ Pneumomediastinum (see Mediastinum)

        ♥ Pneumomediastinum can cause pneumothorax, but pneumothorax cannot cause pneumomediastinum

        ♥ If pneumomediastinum and pneumothorax are seen concurrently, look for the cause of pneumomediastinum as the ultimate cause of the pneumothorax.

    ✓ Pharyngeal, laryngeal, tracheal, or neck trauma

✓ Iatrogenic (only you know what you did!)

✓ May be caused by accidental insertion of pointy sharp object into the lungs.

✓ Iatrogenic causes should especially be sought for pneumomediastinum. This condition may result from the following:

    ✓ Trachea laceration

        ✓ Secondary to endotracheal intubation

        ✓ Occurring during transtracheal wash

✔ Occurring during tracheostomy

✔ Perforation of pharyngeal wall during dentistry

✔ Idiopathic

✔ No trauma or masses can be seen.

✔ Look for bulla formation. Bullae can be seen better after they reinflate in a few days and when viewed on expiratory-phase radiographs.

✔ Some massive chronic pneumothorax are associated with uncommonly minimal clinical signs.

✔ Other cavitated mass lesions

✔ Necrotic neoplasia

✔ Granuloma or abscess

✔ Bronchoesophageal fistula

Types of Pneumothorax

✔ Open: involves direct two-way communication through the chest wall.

✔ Closed: the chest wall is intact, and the damaged lung is the source of air.

✔ Tension pneumothorax: air enters the pleural space during inspiration because of a defect in the lung or the chest wall. Because of a one-way valve effect in the defect, air is trapped during expiration, resulting in positive-pressure air in a pleural space. Ventilation and return of blood to the heart are severely compromised. The radiologic manifestation is a mediastinal shift away from the side of increased intrapleural pressure (see Mediastinal Shift).

Treatment

Treatment involves thoracocentesis, therapy for the underlying disease, and empirical respiratory therapy.

Pleural Effusion

The following are normal conditions or other situations that mimic pleural effusion in cats or dogs:

✓ Pleural fissures

  ✓ In obese patients, excessive fat accumulation sites in the caudal mediastinum, between the right accessory and caudal left lung lobes, may look like a pleural fissure. In such patients, pleural fissures are uncommon.

  ✓ In geriatric patients, pleural fissures may thicken because of fibrosis.

✓ Separation of the lung from the chest wall

  ✓ In obese patients, fat accumulation may appear on the inner aspect of the chest wall (on VD/DV view) or may appear on the suprasternal aspect (on lateral view).

  ✓ Body conformation may also lead to misdiagnosis of pleural effusion (on both projections); you should be especially aware of this in chondrodystrophic dog breeds. Look for:

    ✓ Abnormal costochondral junctions

    ✓ Skin folds superimposed at same level

Physiology of Free Fluid and Radiographic Views

When obtaining and viewing radiographs for possible pleural effusion, keep in mind that fluid falls.

✓ The VD view is the best view for detection of small amounts of pleural effusion because fluid should be placed in the widest part of the chest (that is, dorsally).

  ✓ Allows detection of asymmetrical pleural effusion

  ✓ Provides best view of heart in moderate to severe pleural effusion

  ✋ The VD view may be clinically contraindicated in dyspneic patients

✓ The lateral projection shows fluid accumulation in the interlobar pleural space and reveals separation of the lung from the sternum (Figures 6-2, 6-3, and 6-4).

Roentgen Signs

✓ Lateral projection
  ✓ Pleural fissures
  ✓ Accumulation of ventral soft tissue opacity
✓ DV/VD projection
  ✓ Pleural fissures
  ✓ Opaque layer causing retraction of lung borders away from the ribs
✓ Both views
  ✓ Partial collapse: mild to moderate interstitial lung pattern
  ✓ Complete lobe or lung collapse: alveolar lung pattern
  ♥ Contusion or hemorrhage: focal patchy increased interstitial or alveolar pattern

Pleural Fissures

The following characteristics will help you distinguish fibrosis from fluid:
✓ Fibrosis:
  ✓ The entire length is thin.
  ✓ Appropriate signalment-age, breed, sex, species (occurs more frequently in older dogs than in older cats).
✓ Fluid
  ✓ Appears wedge-shaped on radiograph
  ✓ Widest part of wedge is toward the periphery (that is, away from the lung hilus)
✓ Distribution of fluid
  ✓ With pleural effusion, we assume that the mediastinum is incomplete and that this allows free passage of fluid.
  ✓ Closure can occur secondary to fibrin deposition or occlusion with cells.
✓ Fluid distribution can be symmetrical or asymmetrical:
  ✓ Symmetrical
    ✓ Acute: any fluid type
    ✓ Chronic: water, cells, blood

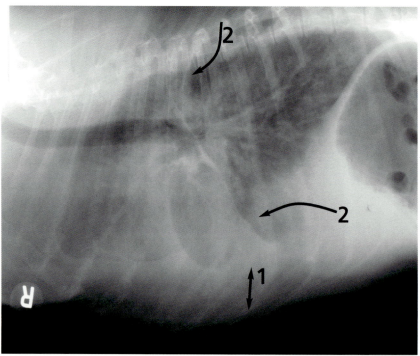

Figure 6-2
Lateral view of a 9 year old male neutered Doberman Pinscher with DCM. Note the increased distance between sternum and lung (1) and pleural fissure lines (2).

✓ Asymmetrical
   ✓ Peracutely: any fluid type
   ✓ Chronic:
      ♥ Chylothorax
      ♥ Pyothorax

♥ Table 6-1 shows commonly associated sequelae of chronic chylothorax (Figure 6-4):

Table 6-1 Sequelae of Chronic Chylothorax

Sequelae	Clinical Relevance
Complete mediastinum	Need to drain both sides for effective therapy
Fibrosing pleuritis	Rigid lungs may not reinflate after fluid drainage
Lung lobe rounding	May be progressive and life-threatening

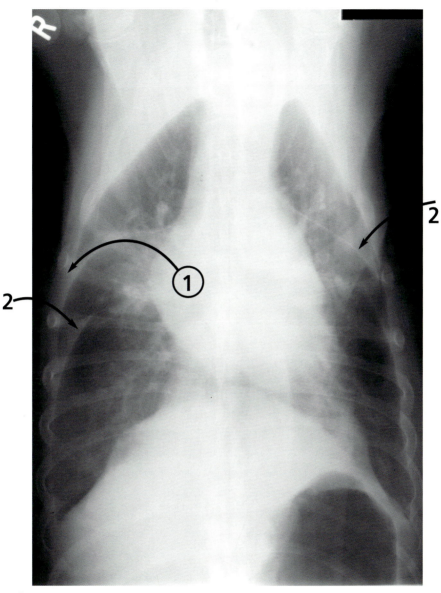

Figure 6-3
Ventrodorsal view of same dog in Figure 6-2. Note retraction of lung borders from body wall (1) and pleural fissure lines (2).

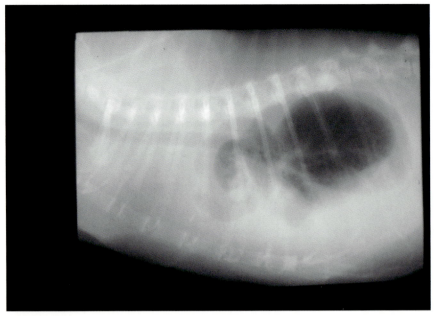

Figure 6-4
Lateral view of 6 year old domestic short haired cat with idiopathic chylothorax. Notice how the lung margins are rounded.

✋ Air (pneumothorax) commonly replaces fluid in the pleural space after drainage (nature really abhors a vacuum!). The source of air infiltration may be the main stem bronchi, lungs, or along the side of the needle. The pneumothorax has no more clinical significance than the original pleural effusion. In the cat, chronic chylothorax is the prognostic equivalent of progressive emphysema in humans.

Pleural Edema

Pleural edema is uncommon, but it does occur. Often, the term is inappropriately used to refer to pleural effusion or pulmonary edema.

✋ Pleural edema is rarely seen with early right-sided or left-sided heart failure in cats.

Types of Fluid

Table 6-2 lists cytologic findings, interpretations of these findings, and conditions in the differential diagnosis.

Table 6-2 Fluid Cytology, Interpretations, and Conditions

Cytology	Interpretation	Differential Diagnois
Blood	Hemorrhage	Trauma, coagulopathy, hemangiosarcoma
Pus	Pyothorax	Foreign body, abscess
Water	Transudate	Right-heart failure, low albumin level, diaphragmatic hernia, vasculitis
Cancer cells	Malignant effusion	Mesothelioma, malignant lymphoma
Chyle	Chylothorax	Idiopathic cause, right-heart failure, cranial mediastinal mass (see Mediastinum)

Testing

After thoracentesis cytologic testing, other tests can be done to definitively diagnose the cause of pleural effusion (Table 6-3).

Table 6-3 Additional Cytologic Testing

Cytology of Pleural Effusion	Additional Testing
Blood	Coagulation panel, platelet count, examination for bleeding
Pus	Culture, drainage/lavage, surgery
Water	Serum chemistry, echocardiography, immunologic testing, abdominal ultrasonography,
Neoplastic cells	Thoracic ultrasonography
Chyle	Echocardiography, measurement of thyroxine, thoracic ultrasonography, angiography

♥ After pleural fluid drainage, radiographs may be used for the following:

✓ To obtain information on the amount of residual fluid.

✓ To detect lesions masked by large amounts of pleural effusion.

✓ To detect any iatrogenic pneumothorax.

✓ To change the course of future testing or therapy.

Concurrent Conditions

✓ Concurrent pneumothorax and pleural effusion may occur together as a result of thoracocentesis; these conditions are rarely concurrent without iatrogenic influences.

✓ Peritoneal and pleural effusion may be concurrent in patients with the following:

- ✓ Neoplasia
- ✓ Right-heart failure
- ✓ Vasculitis
- ✓ Diaphragmatic hernia
- ✓ Coagulopathy

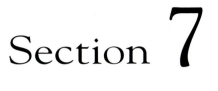

Mediastinum

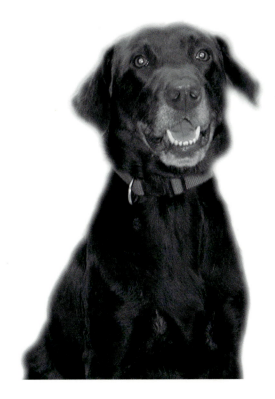

The mediastinum is the space between the two lungs. It contains many vital structures, most of which are radiographically undetectable in normal dogs and cats.

Normal Radiographic Anatomy of the Mediastinum

✓ The mediastinum is usually only a potential space between two layers of mediastinal pleura.

✓ In most normal dogs and cats, the mediastinum is incomplete; fluid can freely traverse between the left and right pleural spaces.

Normal Visible Structures

✓ Cranial mediastinum
  ✓ Trachea: air is seen in the lumen and mucosal border
  ✓ Thymus: visible only in neonates
  ✓ Lymph nodes, esophagus, and serosal margins of trachea are occult
✓ Middle mediastinum
  ✓ Heart and aortic arch
  ✓ Tracheobronchial lymph nodes and esophagus are occult
✓ Caudal mediastinum
  ✓ Descending aorta
  ✓ Caudal vena cava
  ✓ Esophagus is occult

Mediastinal Reflections

✓ Cranial mediastinum
  ✓ On ventrodorsal (VD)/dorsalventro (DV) views, the cranial mediastinum appears as a diagonal line
  ✓ Orientation is from cranial right to caudal left
  ✓ Represents the normal location and orientation of the thymus
  ✓ Allows the cranial tip of the left cranial lung lobe to

extend into the thorax on, or to the right of, the midline.

✓ Allows the caudal medial part of the right cranial lobe to wrap around the cranial ventral aspect of the heart and extend to the left of midline.

✓ The ventral aspect is at the level of the sternal lymph node.

♥ Fills with fat in obese patients (dogs and cats):

  ♥ VD/DV projection: mimics a mass

  ♥ Lateral projection: the separated lung lobe apices may mimic bullae, bubbles of free air, or pleural effusion.

✓ Caudal mediastinum

Between right accessory and left caudal lobes

✓ VD/DV projection: a straight line between heart apex and diaphragm.

✓ Occult on lateral projections

♥ Fills with fat in obese patients (dogs and cats)

♥ VD/DV projection: mimics a pleural effusion

Mediastinal Diseases

Pneumomediastinum

On radiograph (Figure 7-1), you can see structures that are normally occult

✓ Serosal border of trachea

✓ Adventitial (outer) border of the esophagus

✓ Brachycephalic trunk, left subclavian, and cranial vena cava

♥ There are three sources of the air found in pneumomediastinum

1. Ruptured tubes:

  ♥ Trachea

  ✓ Esophagus

2. Seepage into cranial or caudal mediastinum:

  ♥ Deep fascial planes of the neck, pharynx, or larynx

  ✓ Retroperitoneum space

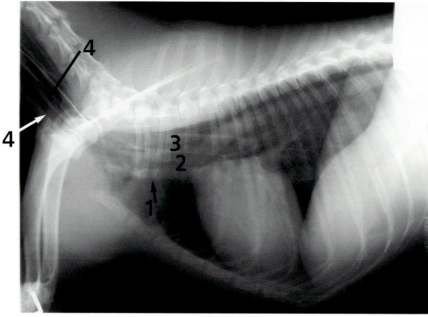

Figure 7-1
Pneumomediastinum. You can see the distinct cranial vena cava (1), brachycephalic trunk (2), both mucosal and serosal margins of the trachea (3), and air in the deep fascial planes of the neck (4).

3. Lungs or bugs

✓ Lung trauma has occurred, but visceral pleura is intact

✓ Emphysematous mediastinitis

♥ Uncomplicated pneumomediastinum is not clinically significant, but the condition can cause a secondary pneumothorax (see Pleural Space Diseases).

♥ Additional testing can be done; the easiest involves looking for neck trauma. Pneumomediastinum is often associated with traumatic placement of a tracheal tube.

♥ Therapy can involve treatment of the underlying cause or the secondary pneumothorax.

Mediastinal Masses

Cranial Mediastinum

✓ General radiographic signs

    ✓ Lateral projection

✓ Dorsal displacement of the trachea
  ♥ Beware the undulating trachea caused in normal dogs and cats by neck flexion
  ♥ Also seen with pleural effusion
  ♥ Not seen with fat in the cranial mediastinum
  ✓ Rounding of ventral mediastinal border. (Note in Figure 7-1 the straight line of the ventral border of the cranial vena cava.

✓ VD/DV projection
  ✓ Widening of the cranial mediastinum
  ♥ Left and right borders have convex shape.
  ♥ Fat usually has parallel, straight borders.

✓ Causes
  ✓ Megaesophagus: (dorsal location)
    🖐 Ventral deviation of trachea
  ✓ Cranial mediastinal lymph nodes (Figures 7-2 and 7-3).
    ✓ Ventral deviation of the normal ventral border (in the same location as the cranial vena cava).
    ✓ Malignant or reactive disease
      ♥ Primary disease site
        ✓ Head or neck
        ✓ Thorax
        ✓ Disseminated disease
  ✓ Thymus (middle to ventral)
    ✓ Lateral projection shows dorsal displacement of the trachea.
      ✓ Mass often seems to wrap around cranial heart border
    ✓ Thymic lymphoma or thymoma (Figures 7-4 and 7-5)
  ✓ Ectopic thyroid mass (middle)
  ✓ Nerve root tumor (dorsal)
  ✓ Sternal lymph node (ventral); visible on lateral projection (Figure 7-2)
    ✓ Soft tissue mass dorsal to second sternebra in dogs
    ✓ Often more caudal in cats
  ✓ VD/DV projection

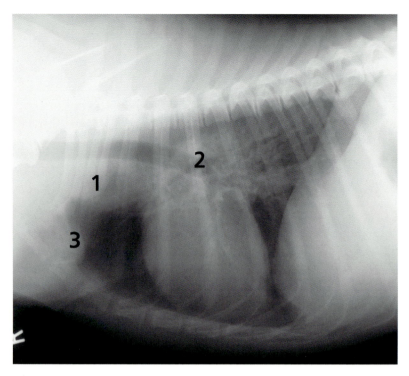

Figure 7-2

Lateral view of 5 year old female spayed Golden Retriever with lymphoma. Note the increased opacity associated with enlarged cranial mediastinal (1), tracheobronchial (2), and sternal (3) lymph nodes.

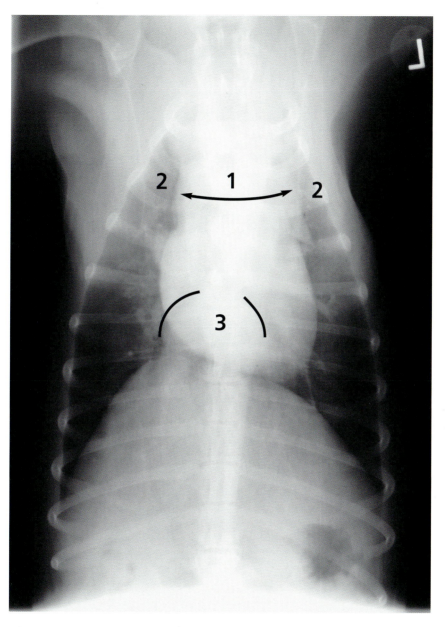

Figure 7-3

In the same patient as Figure 7-2, you can also see the increased width (1) of the cranial mediastinum with convex-shaped rounded margins (2), and the increased opacity in the caudal heart base with abaxial displacement of the caudal mainstem bronchi (3).

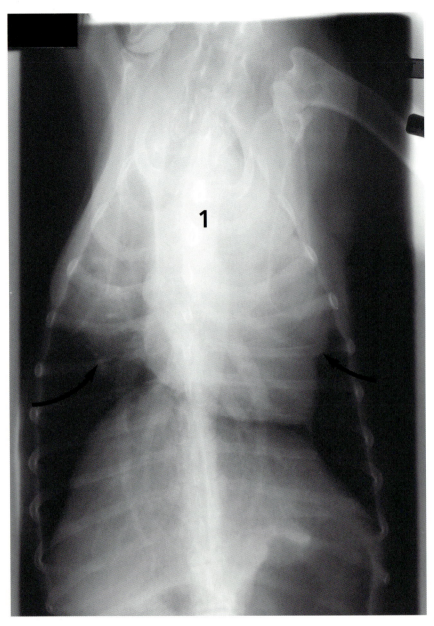

Figure 7-4
Dorsoventral view of 12 year old female spayed Dalmation with thymoma.
Note the large cranial mediastinal mass (1) causing bilateral caudal
displacement of the cranial lung lobes (arrows).

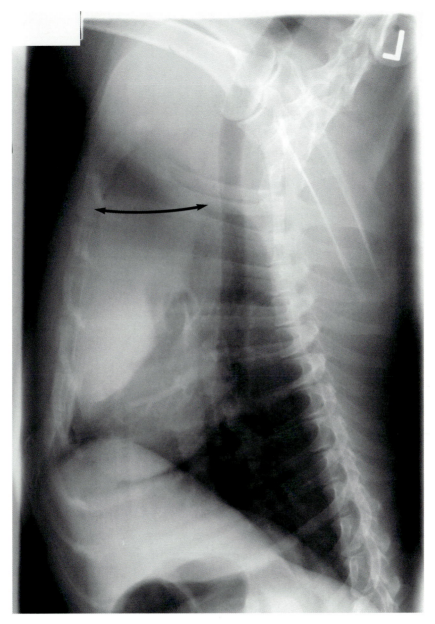

Figure 7-5
Lateral view of same dog as in Figure 7-4. Note the dorsal displacement of the trachea and caudal displacement of the cranial lung lobes by a large cranial mediastinal mass (arrow).

✓ Occult or mild widening
✓ Malignant or reactive
  ♥ Primary disease site
    ♥ Cranial abdomen (stomach, pancreas, liver)
    ✓ Mammary chain (first 2 or 3 pairs of glands)
    ✓ Disseminated disease (lymphoma, fungal)
♥ Bronchial cysts (cats) (ventral)
  ✓ Proximal or in apposition to cranial heart border

Middle Mediastinum

✓ General radiographic signs
  ✓ Lateral and VD/DV projections:
    ♥ Displacement of mainstem bronchi or tracheal bifurcation
  ✓ Megaesophagus
  ✓ Tracheobronchial lymph nodes (Figures 7-2 and 7-3)
    ✓ Cranial to the cranial left and right mainstem bronchi
    ✓ Caudal to (that is, between) the caudal mainstem bronchi
    ✓ Lateral projection
      ♥ Caudal node
      ♥ Dorsal or ventral deviation of tracheal bifurcation
    ✓ Malignant or reactive
      ♥ Primary disease site
        ♥ Thorax, primary lung neoplasia
        ✓ Disseminated disease, lymphoma, fungal

Caudal Mediastinum

✓ Megaesophagus
✓ Stomach herniation (see Section 8)

Disorders of the Esophagus

✓ Megaesophagus (Figures 7-6 and 7-7)
General radiographic signs

- ✔ Ventral deviation of trachea
- ✔ Appearance of thin opaque lines representing the walls of the air-filled esophagus
- ✔ Regional increased soft tissue opacity representing fluid-filled esophagus
- ✔ Focal location

In the cranial mediastinum, megaesophagus may be caused by the following:

- ✔ Vascular ring anomaly
- ✔ Redundancy (normal in Bulldog = diverticulum)
- ✔ Stricture or foreign body

In the caudal mediastinum, megaesophagus may be caused by the following:

- ✔ Esophagitis
- ✔ Stricture or foreign body
- ✔ Stomach herniation

- ✔ General localized

Causes include the following:

- ♥ Idiopathic
- ♥ Low tone (as a result of anesthesia, obtunded condition)
- ♥ Aerophagia
- ✔ Myasthenia gravis
- ✔ Esophagitis
- 🖑 Seemingly endless list of endocrine, toxic, immune, degenerative, neoplastic, metabolic, traumatic, and inflammatory causes that are beyond the scope of this text.

Disorders of the Trachea

Hypoplasia

- ✔ Common in brachycephalic breeds
- ✔ Very small in English Bulldogs
  - ✔ You must determine whether the radiographic appearance represents a normal variant or hypoplasia.
  - ♥ The following concurrent diseases exacerbate hypoplasia:
    - ✔ Overly long and thickened soft palate

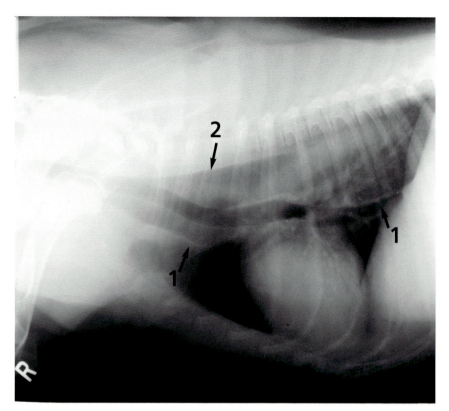

Figure 7-6
Lateral view of 5 year old male Chesapeake Bay retriever with megae-sophagus. Note ventral (1) and dorsal (2) margins of diluted esophagus and ventral deviation of trachea.

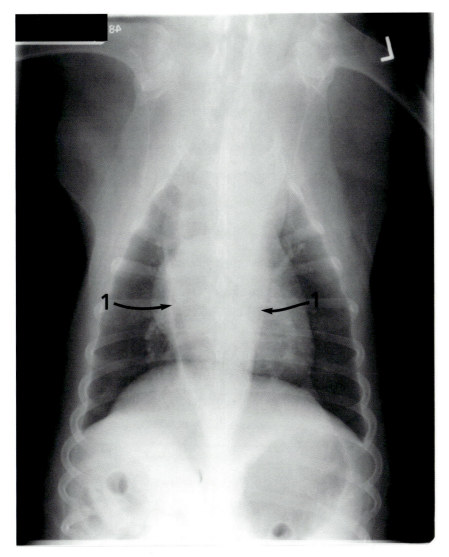

Figure 7-7

Megaesophagus. Dorsal ventral view of same dog as Figure 7-6. Note borders of dilated esophagus (1).

✔ Stenotic nares

✋ The hypoplastic trachea is rigid and does not dynamically collapse

Tracheal Collapse (Figures 7-8, 7-9, and 7-10)

✔ Caused by internal defect (weakness) or external compression

✔ Characterized by loss of rigidity

    ✔ Entire wall collapses

    ✔ Dorsal tracheal muscle folds into lumen

♥ Associated breeds and diseases

    ♥ Toy breeds

    ♥ Obesity

    ♥ Bronchitis (this may be a cause or an effect)

Static Collapse

✔ Left atrial enlargement at the level of tracheal bifurcation (Figure 7-8)

✔ Severe loss of rigidity

Dynamic Collapse (Figures 7-9 and 7-10)

✔ Extrathoracic (neck or thoracic inlet)

    ✔ Collapses on inspiration

    ✔ Commonly seen on routine inspiration-phase lateral projections

✔ Intrathoracic (thoracic inlet or intrathoracic)

    ✔ Collapses on expiration (see Figure 7-9)

    ✔ May be seen on routine expiration-phase lateral projections

Mediastinal Shift

Mediastinal shift occurs when midline structures (heart, mediastinal fat) are displaced to a side. This may be caused by masses which push the structures or by diseases that are associated with reduced size which pull the structures.

Masses

    ✔ Lung or other masses that expand beyond normal size

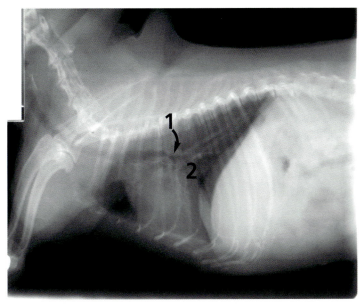

Figure 7-8
Static left mainstem bronchial narrowing (collapse) (1) due to compression by an enlarged left atrium (2).

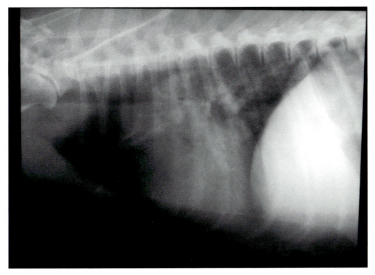

Figure 7-9
Lateral expiratory phase view of 14 year old female spayed Cocker Spaniel showing collapse of the caudal trachea and main stem bronchi.

✔ Asymmetrical pleural disease (caused by air or effusion)

  ♥ Tension pneumothorax (see Section 6 on pleural disease)

✔ Unilateral or lobar hyperinflation; look for physiologic or post-lobectomy reasons for hyperinflation.

  ✔ Lobes may be adjacent to chronic atelectasis

  ✔ Pathologic: partial/dynamic bronchial obstruction

Diseases of reduced size

  ♥ Atelectasis of one or more lobes in a lung

  ✔ Seen commonly when animals are under general anesthesia

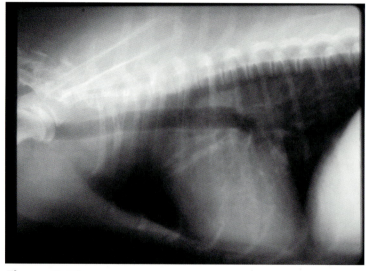

Figure 7-10
Lateral inspiratory phase radiograph of same dog as Figure 7-9. Note normal size of trachea and mainstem bronchi.

Section 8

Diaphragm

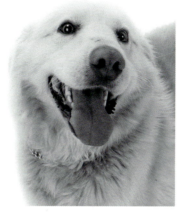

The diaphragm is the structure that separates life in the thorax from a peritoneal existence. Although taken for granted as a dynamic intact structure, it causes many problems when traumatized or as a consequence of faulty development.

Normal Radiographic Features

The diaphragm consists of two parts: the cupula and the crura.

Cupula

The cupula is the central tendon region of the diaphragm and is considered the cranial ventral "dome."

✔ On VD/DV view, the cranial-most part is usually slightly right of midline.

Left and Right Crura

The crura are the dorsal muscular portions of the diaphragm.

✔ They originate from the third and fourth lumbar vertebrae

✔ Gastric fundus resides immediately caudal to left crus

✔ The caudal vena cava enters the right crus.

The following are common changes seen as a consequence of positioning in dogs:

✔ Right lateral view: right crus cranial to left crus

✔ Left lateral view: left crus cranial to right crus

✔ VD view: both crura are seen distinctly in addition to cupula

✔ DV view: Only the cupula is seen; crura are occult

Special considerations in cats include the following:

♥ The movement of the crura on lateral views is much less dependable than in dogs.

♥ During hyperinflation, "tenting" can be seen.

✔ Look for stretching between sites of rib attachment.

Radiographic Features of Hernia

Congenital Hernia

Three types of congenital hernia are peritoneal pericardial diaphragmatic hernia, hiatal hernia, and congenital diaphragmatic hernia. The findings of the latter condition are the same as those for traumatic hernia (see following discussion).

♥ Peritoneal pericardial diaphragmatic hernia (Figures 8-1 and 8-2)

   ✓ Always congenital

   ✓ Usually an incidental finding

   ✓ Often associated with umbilical hernia or pectus excavatum

   ♥ Clinical signs occur when organs, especially the liver, become entrapped. Entrapment leads to pericardial effusion or necrosis.

   ♥ Mimics a huge heart or pericardial effusion

   ♥ On lateral projection, classic radiographic finding is dorsal peritoneopericardial mesothelial remnant

✓ Hiatal hernia

   ♥ Occurs intermittently

   ♥ Chinese Shar-peis are predisposed.

   ✓ Contrast radiography is needed for diagnosis (along with lucky timing).

      ✓ Typical finding is rugal folds in the chest (Figure 8-3).

   ✓ Often associated with regional megaesophagus

Traumatic Diaphragmatic Hernia

(Figures 8-4 and 8-5)

✓ Usually a right ventral defect

✓ Commonly due to abdominal or pelvic trauma (e.g., car accident).

✓ Herniation of abdominal viscera can range from mild to massive and can affect any of the following:

   ✓ Peritoneal fat

   ♥ Liver

   ♥ Intestines

   ✓ Almost anything in the abdomen

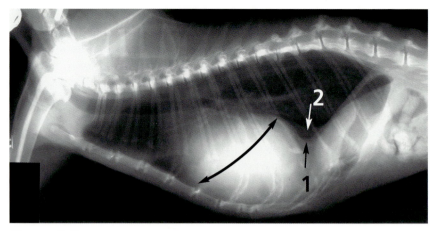

Figure 8-1
Lateral view of 18 year old female spayed domestic short hair with Pericardial peritoneal diaphragmatic hernia. Note increased size of cardiac silhouette (arrow), mesothelial remnant (1) ventral to caudal vena cava (2).

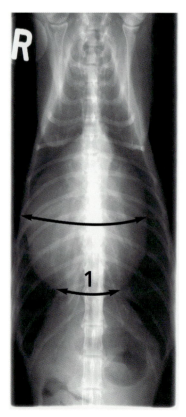

Figure 8-2
Ventral dorsal view of the same patient as Figure 8-1, note silhouetting of the diaphragm (1) with enlarged cardiac margin (arrow).

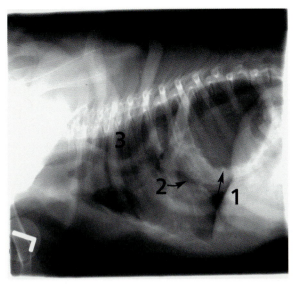

Figure 8-3
Lateral view of 4 month old female Shar Pei with Hiatal hernia. Rugal folds of the gastric fundus (1) can be seen in the chest. The border of stomach is outlined (2), and a secondary megaesophagus is noted (3).

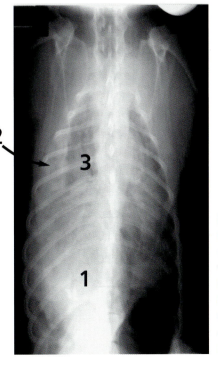

Figure 8-4
Dorsal ventral view of 2 year old male neutered mix-breed dog with traumatic diaphragmatic hernia. The silhouette sign between the heart and diaphragm (1), air-filled bowel loops in the chest 2), and the retraction of lung margins (3) are visible.

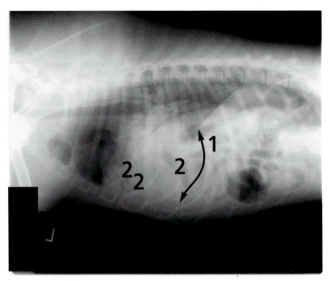

Figure 8-5
Lateral view of same patient as Figure 8-4, this view shows the silhouette sign between heart and diaphragm (1) and the bowel loops in the chest (2).

✓ The clinical significance of the hernia is proportional to the volume of abdominal viscera in the collapsing lung and is inversely proportional to the diameter of the defect. A defect with a smaller diameter is more likely to lead to entrapment, strangulation, necrosis, and effusion.

✓ Herniation is easiest to diagnose when air-filled intestines enter the thorax. Diagnosis is most difficult when soft tissue or fat structures herniate.

Rare Hernia

✓ Gastroesophageal intussusception

✓ Paraesophageal hernia

✓ Eventration of the diaphragm

Reasons for Loss of Diaphragmatic Border

✓ Focal findings include
- ♥ Alveolar lung pattern
- ✓ Lung mass touching diaphragm
- ✓ Focal pleural effusion
- ✓ Hernia

✓ Generalized findings include
- ♥ Pleural effusion
- ✓ Large hernia

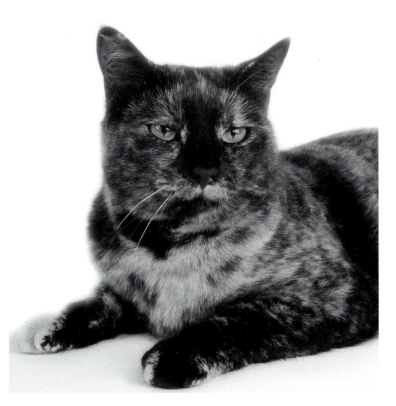

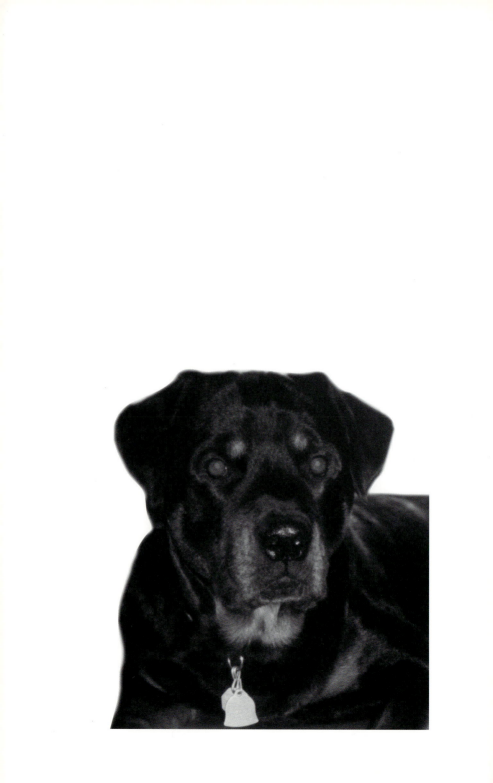

Section 9

Body Wall and Ribs

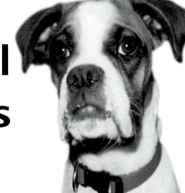

Body Wall

Body conformation varies widely among dog breeds. In cats, conformation is much more consistent.

Normal Variations

Ribs

✔ Ribs are much wider ventrally in many dog breeds.

✔ Rib margins may mimic a pleural fissure or margins of a mass.

✔ Variations in number of ribs (12 or 14 pairs) are incidental.

✔ Some notable features of costochondral junctions and costal arches include the following:

  ✔ In Basset Hounds, the junctions and arches are dramatic on the ventro-dorsal (VD)/dorsal-ventro (DV) view.

  ✔ In older dogs and cats, they mimic nodules.

  ✔ In neonates, they are flexible and can lead to flail chest (see under Radiographic Appearance of Disease) with rib fractures.

  ✋ They are never the site of neoplasia (ribs– yes; cartilage– no).

Spine

✔ Spondylosis deformans is common in older dogs and cats.

✔ Hemivertebrae are common in brachycephalic breeds of dogs.

✔ The disk space between T10 and T11 is normally narrowed (also referred to as anticlinal space).

Sternum

✔ Bridging degenerative changes similar to spondylosis deformans, are common in older dogs and cats, and are clinically incidental.

✔ Deformities of sternebrae are usually incidental.

  ✔ One type of deformity is pectus excavatum:
    ✔ Dorsal deviation of caudal sternebrae
    ✔ Displaced heart off of the midline (mediastinal shift)
    ♥ Commonly associated with pericardial peritoneal diaphragmatic hernia (see Diaphragm)

  ✔ Other anomalies include abnormal shape and number of sternebrae.

Skin and Other Parts of Body Wall

✓ Nipples are inconsistently seen.

✓ Ticks, dirt, and other debris are visible and can mimic lung nodules.

✓ Excessive skin folds are common in many dog breeds.

✓ The following radiographic considerations should be kept in mind:

    ✓ Soft tissue "lesions" are seen best on nondependent skin surfaces (e.g., nipples are most often seen superimposed on the lung on VD projection).

    ♥ When suspicious nodules are present, mark external lumps, bumps, and nipples. Place a small amount of barium paste or a small metallic marker, such as a washer or pellet. Then repeat the radiographs.

Radiographic Appearance of Disease

Ribs

Radiographic Techniques for Evaluating Ribs

♥ VD/DV projection is more valuable than lateral projections.

✋ Turn radiograph upside down: doing so allows you to concentrate on ribs and pay less attention to the heart, lungs, and other structures.

♥ Look for any asymmetry

Fractures (Figure 9-1)

✓ Commonly secondary to blunt trauma

✓ Commonly associated with pneumothorax

✓ Marked by flail chest, in which the body wall moves paradoxically with the phase of ventilation (inward during inspiration and outward with expiration).

♥ Fracture may exacerbate lung trauma and ventilatory pain.

✓ In adults, multiple fractures may occur in adjacent ribs.

♥ In neonates, single fractures in adjacent ribs (due to flexible costochondral junctions).

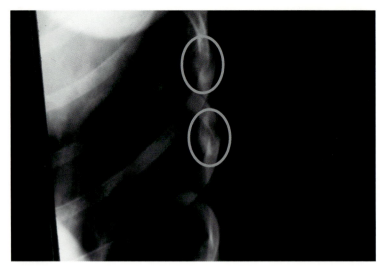

Figure 9-1

Pathological fracture of ribs due to multiple myeloma. Note lysis and irregular shape of fracture fragment margins, indicating a pathological process. Image has been intentionally printed up-side down.

Neoplasia

✓ The ribs are a common site of primary and metastatic neoplasia.

✓ Primary neoplasia

   ✓ Chondrosarcoma is most common (Figure 9-2).

   ✓ Neoplasms commonly invade adjacent soft tissues and other ribs.

   ✓ Distal rib is commonly affected (neoplasms develop near, not in, the costochondral junction).

   ♥ Neoplasms more commonly extend inward than outward. They may not be apparent on palpation and may have a large intrathoracic component.

   ✓ The following are radiographic signs of primary rib neoplasia:

      ♥ Asymmetry

         ✓ Increased width of intercostal space

         ✓ Irregular or fuzzy rib margins

      ✓ Changes in opacity (lysis or proliferation)

      ✓ Pathological fractures

      ♥ Extrapleural mass sign

♥ Broad-based toward chest wall
✓ Metastatic neoplasia
  ✓ Characterized by focal lytic or sclerotic changes.
  ✓ Multiple ribs are often affected.
  ♥ Commonly the dog or cat presents with signs referable to pathologic fracture of affected ribs.
  ✓ The extrapleural mass sign is less common than with primary neoplasia, and the masses are rarely as large.

Infectious Disease
✓ Geographic predilections

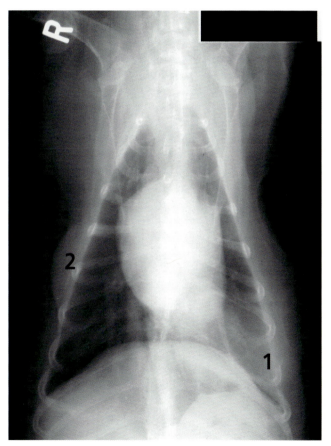

Figure 9-2
Rib chondrosarcoma. Note lysis of rib (1), and incidental bodywall lipoma on the right side (2).

✓ Characterized by lytic or sclerotic changes

✓ Often associated with draining tracts

Spine

Note that the scope of this discussion is limited; see Recommended Readings.

Intervertebral Disk Disease

✓ Affects disk spaces between T10 and T11 and caudally

✓ Clinically relevant signs include

    ✓ Narrowed disk space

        ✓ Smaller intervertebral foramen

        ✓ Focal increased opacity in intervertebral foramen

        ✓ Mineralization of disk material in the disk space is often incidental.

Discospondylitis

✓ This condition is not the same as spondylosis deformans (see preceding discussion). It is characterized by inflammation of the end plates of adjacent vertebrae.

✓ The following are typical radiographic signs:

    ♥ Acute: no signs (condition is occult)

    ♥ Subacute: focal lysis of adjacent end plates

    ✓ Chronic: sclerosis surrounding lytic regions

Neoplasia

✓ Primary and metastatic neoplasms are common.

✓ Characterized by regional lysis or sclerosis

♥ Very subtle in the dorsal, often overexposed, portions of the thoracic radiograph. As a result, very intensive scrutiny with bright light is necessary.

✋ Metastatic neoplasia seems to occur frequently in T3.

✓ Specific neoplasias:

    ✓ Osteosarcoma: most common primary tumor; also common as a metastatic lesion (Figure 9-3)

    ✓ Myeloma

        Classic: multiple areas of discrete focal round lysis

        Common: regional lysis or sclerosis

✓ Nerve root tumors

  ✓ Unilateral lysis, adjacent to foramen

  ✓ Affects C6 to T3

Sternum

✓ Degenerative changes may appear aggressive.

✓ Neoplasia and infection are uncommon.

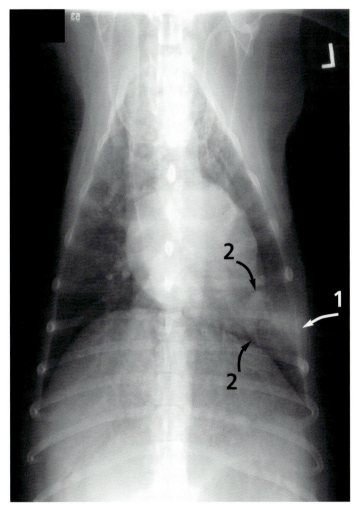

Figure 9-3
Metastatic osteosarcoma in the rib. This view (DV) shows lysis of the rib (1). The curvilinear convex-shaped margins at the area of increased opacity indicates the extrapleural sign–a mass of the bodywall or in the pleural space (2).

✓ When infection occurs, draining tracts are common.

✓ Pectus excavatum is associated with pericardial peritoneal diaphragmatic hernia.

Other Body Wall Diseases

✓ Trauma
  ✓ Hematoma
  ✓ Deep fascial-plane and subcutaneous air (mimics pneumothorax)

✓ Neoplasia
  ✓ Lipoma (see Figure 9-2)
  ✓ Fibrosarcoma in cats (especially vaccine-associated)

Appendices

A. Technique Chart

Example Thoracic Technique Chart

WITH GRID

CM	11	12	13	14	15
KVP	80	83	86	89	92

.8 mAs
100 mA x 1/120 sec

FAST SCREENS

CM	16	17	18	19	20	21	22	23	24	25	26	27	28	29	30
KVP	87	90	93	96	98	101	105	109	113	117	121	111	113	117	121

1.7 mAs
100 mA x 1/60 sec

2.5 mAs
300 mA x 1/120sec

TABLE TOP (NON- GRID)   DETAIL SCREENS

CM	5	6	7	8	9	10	11	12	13	14	15
KVP	54	56	58	60	62	64	66	68	70	72	74

2.5 mAs
300 mA x 1/120 sec

B. Lateral Thorax Positioning

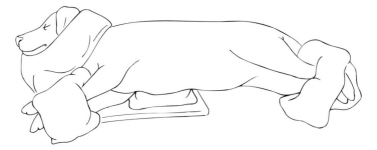

1. Measure animal at widest point (12th or 13th rib)
2. Choose a cassette size that fits the animal's thorax
3. Make sure the animal is in a "true" lateral position, not obliqued
4. Pull front legs forward

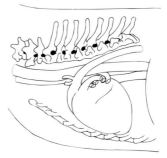

5. Center beam at caudal border of scapula
6. Include sternum in primary beam
7. Take radiograph at peak inspiration

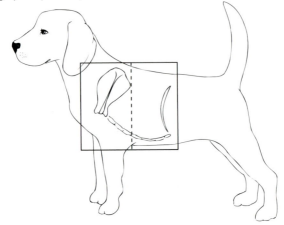

C. Ventral-Dorsal Thorax Positioning

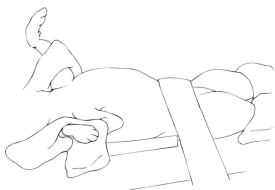

1. Measure the animal at the tallest point (11th or 12th rib)
2. Choose a cassette that fits the animal's thorax
3. Place animal in dorsal recumbency
4. Make sure animal is straight, not obliqued
5. Include thorax from the manubrium to the 13th rib
6. Take exposure at peak inspiration

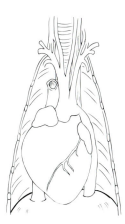

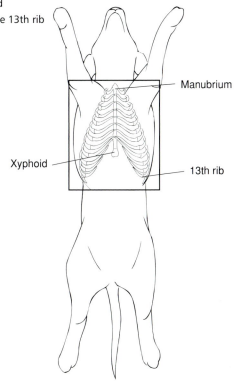

Manubrium

Xyphoid

13th rib

D. Dorsal Ventral Positioning

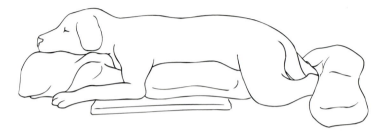

1. Measure the animal at the tallest point (11th or 12th rib)
2. Choose a cassette that fits the animal's thorax
3. Place animal in ventral recumbency
4. Make sure animal is straight, not obliqued
5. Include thorax from the manubrium to the 13th rib
6. Take exposure at peak inspiration

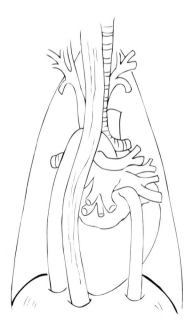

We hope you enjoy this **Made Easy** Series volume.
If you would like more information on **Made Easy** Series products
please call 877-306-9793 or visit us at www.tetonnm.com

NO POSTAGE
NECESSARY
IF MAILED
IN THE
UNITED STATES

BUSINESS REPLY MAIL

FIRST-CLASS MAIL   PERMIT NO.29   JACKSON, WY

POSTAGE WILL BE PAID BY ADDRESSEE

Teton NewMedia
P.O. Box 4833
Jackson, WY 83001-9965